Emergency
Ultrasound
Made Easy

For Elsevier:

Commissioning Editor: Laurence Hunter
Development Editor: Helen Leng
Project Manager: Caroline Horton
Designer: Erik Bigland
Illustration Manager: Bruce Hogarth

Emergency Ultrasound Made Easy

Justin Bowra MBBS FACEM

Director of Emergency Medicine Training
Department of Emergency Medicine
Liverpool Hospital
Sydney
Australia

Russell E McLaughlin MB FRCSI FFAEM MMedSci

Consultant in Emergency Medicine
Ulster Hospital
Belfast
UK

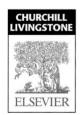

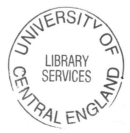

EDINBURGH LONDON NEW YORK OXFORD PHILADELPHIA ST LOUIS SYDNEY
TORONTO 2006

**CHURCHILL
LIVINGSTONE**
ELSEVIER

© 2006, Elsevier Limited. All rights reserved.

The right of Justin Bowra and Russell E McLaughlin to be identified as authors of this work has been asserted by them in accordance with the Copyright, Designs and Patents Act 1988.

First edition 2006

ISBN-13 9780443101507
ISBN-10 0443101507

British Library Cataloguing in Publication Data
A catalogue record for this book is available from the British Library

Library of Congress Cataloging in Publication Data
A catalog record for this book is available from the Library of Congress

Note
Neither the publisher nor the editors assume any responsibility for any loss or injury and/or damage to persons or property arising out of or related to any use of the material contained in this book. It is the responsibility of the treating practitioner, relying on independent expertise and knowledge of the patient, to determine the best treatment and method of application for the patient.

The Publisher

Printed in China

Contents

Contributors

Dr Roslyn Bell BSc MRCS FRCR
Specialist Registrar in Radiology
Royal Victoria Hospital
Belfast, UK

Dr Justin Bowra MBBS FACEM
Director of Emergency Medicine Training
Department of Emergency Medicine
Liverpool Hospital, Sydney, Australia

Mr Niall Collum MRCSE
Specialist Registrar in Emergency
Medicine, Belfast City Hospital
Belfast, UK

Dr Fergal Cummins
Emergency Registrar, Terenure
Dublin, Eire

Dr Michael Hyland FRCR
Consultant Radiologist, Ulster Hospital
Belfast, UK

Dr Anthony P Joseph FACEM
Emergency Physician, Royal North
Shore Hospital,
Lecturer, Faculty of Medicine, University
of Sydney, Australia

Dr Sabrina Kuah FRANZCOG
Consultant Obstetrician and
Gynaecologist
Pebble Bay, Singapore

Dr Stella McGinn PhD FRACP MRCPE
Staff Specialist in Nephrology
Royal North Shore Hospital,
Clinical Senior Lecturer, Department
of Medicine
Northern Clinical School, University of
Sydney, Australia

Mr Sean J McGovern FFAEM FRCSI
Consultant in Emergency Medicine
Ulster Hospital
Belfast, UK

Mr Russell E McLaughlin MB FRCSI FFAEM
MMedSci
Consultant in Emergency Medicine
Ulster Hospital
Belfast, UK

Mr Charles J Martyn BScHons FRCSI FFAEM
Consultant in Emergency Medicine and
Clinical Director Specialist Surgery
Ulster Hospital, Belfast, UK

Dr George Robert Rudan MBBS FRACP
Consultant Physician, Cardiologist
Manly Hospital
Sydney, Australia

Dr Peter K Thompson BSc FRCS FFAEM FACEM
Consultant in Emergency Medicine
King's College Hospital
London, UK

Dr R E Richard Wright MPhil FFRRCSI FRCR
Consultant Radiologist, Ulster Hospital
Clinical Director, Clinical Diagnostics
Directorate
Belfast, UK

Preface

Ultrasound (US) is a safe, rapid imaging technique. It is non-invasive and painless and it is used widely by radiologists, cardiologists (echocardiography) and obstetricians. However, its use in emergency medicine is a more recent phenomenon.

Emergency US is used to answer very specific questions, such as the presence or absence of AAA (abdominal aortic aneurysm), or of free fluid (such as blood) in the abdomen after trauma. Unlike other imaging modalities (e.g. CT scan) it is a rapid technique that can 'come to the patient'.

Emergency US is *not* a substitute for formal US by an appropriately trained radiologist. It has no role in routine situations such as antenatal screening. Its role in some areas (such as urgent diagnosis of paediatric fractures) is still evolving, and future editions of the book will reflect this.

Emergency Ultrasound Made Easy is aimed particularly at specialists and trainees in emergency medicine, surgery and intensive care. However, its scope is broad. For example, rapid diagnosis of DVT (deep vein thrombosis) may be of interest to any hospital doctor, and central venous cannulation is vital in operating theatres.

There are already many excellent comprehensive textbooks of ultrasound, and this book is not designed as such. As the only pocket-sized handbook of emergency US, this book provides a rapid guide to its use and interpretation. It is designed to be accessible and easy to use in an urgent situation (e.g. a shocked trauma patient).

Justin Bowra & Russell McLaughlin

Acknowledgements

To our wives Stella McGinn and Ros Bell whose patience and good humour made this possible!

Thanks to Dr Sanjeeva Abeywickrema, Consultant Radiologist, St Georges Hospital, Sydney.

Abbreviations

Note. Many abbreviations are not standardized. For example, 'artery' may be abbreviated to A or a; 'free fluid' to FF, ff, f or f.f.; 'right internal jugular vein' to rij or RIJV; and 'right kidney' to Rk or rk.)

A	artery
AAA	abdominal aortic aneurysm
AP	anteroposterior
ARF	acute renal failure
ASIS	anterior superior iliac spine
ATLS®	Advanced Trauma Life Support
bl	bladder
CBD	common bile duct
CCA	common carotid artery
CCF	congestive cardiac failure
CPD	continuous professional development
CPR	cardiopulmonary resuscitation
CT	computed tomography
CVC	central vein cannula
CXR	chest X-ray
DDH	developmental dysplasia of hip
DPL	diagnostic peritoneal lavage
DVT	deep vein thrombosis
EBU	emergency bedside ultrasound
ED	Emergency Department
EP	ectopic pregnancy
FAST	focused abdominal sonography in trauma *or* focused assessment with sonography in trauma
f.b.	foreign body
FB	foreign body
ff	free fluid
FF	free fluid
FV	femoral vein
GA	gestational age
GB	gallbladder
IJV	internal jugular vein
IUP	*in utero* pregnancy
IVC	inferior vena cava
li	liver
LMP	last menstrual period
LS	longitudinal section
LV	left ventricle (or left ventricular)
MSD	mean sac diameter
NICE	National Institute for Clinical Excellence
OT	operating theatre
PCKD	polycystic kidney disease
PE	pulmonary embolism or embolus
PEA	pulseless electrical activity
PEEP	positive end-expiratory pressure
PZT	piezo-electric transducer
rij	right internal jugular vein
rijv	right internal jugular vein
Rk	right kidney
RV	right ventricle (or right ventricular)
SCFE	slipped capital femoral epiphysis
SCM	sternocleidomastoid muscle
SMA	superior mesenteric artery
SOB	short of breath
SPC	suprapubic catheter
TA	transabdominal
TS	transverse section
TV	transvaginal
TVS	transvaginal ultrasound
US	ultrasound
V	vein
vb	vertebral body
WES	wall-echo shadow

Chapter 1

Introduction

Justin Bowra

What is ultrasound?

Diagnostic ultrasound (US) is a safe, rapid imaging technique. It is non-invasive and painless, requires no contrast media and no special patient preparation. US is used widely by radiologists, cardiologists (echocardiography) and obstetricians. However, it is only in recent years that its role has emerged in the field of emergency medicine. (See Ch. 2: *How ultrasound works.*)

What is emergency US?

Emergency US, also known as emergency bedside ultrasound (EBU), limited US or focused US, is a modification of US performed by non-radiologists such as emergency physicians and surgeons. Unlike other imaging modalities (e.g. CT scan) it is a rapid technique that can 'come to the patient' and be repeated as often as necessary.

It allows rapid bedside identification of certain life-threatening conditions such as:

✔ abdominal aortic aneurysm (AAA);
✔ traumatic haemoperitoneum (FAST scan: focused abdominal sonography in trauma);
✔ pericardial tamponade.

It also improves the safety of certain procedures by allowing them to be performed under real-time guidance, such as:

1. central vein cannulation;
2. drainage of pericardial tamponade;
3. soft tissue foreign body removal;
4. suprapubic catheter insertion.

What it isn't (you are not a radiologist!)

Unlike formal ultrasound, this technique does not require years of training. Studies have shown that it can be quickly taught and that as few as ten scans may suffice for an operator to obtain acceptable scans for a given indication. (See Ch. 14: *Getting trained and staying trained.*)

However, it must be emphasized that it is **not** a substitute for formal US by an appropriately trained radiologist. It has no role in routine situations such as antenatal screening or the diagnosis of breast lumps, for example.

Why is this? Radiologists are trained to scan and interpret images in detail, using an in-depth understanding of the relevant anatomy, pathology and US images of the scanned area. By contrast, emergency US is limited to answering **specific** questions only, and training and credentialing guidelines reflect this (Ch. 14).

First considerations

It is wise to bear in mind the following important principles when training in emergency US:

Table 1.1 Binary thinking

Clinical situation	The right question (answer: yes or no)	The wrong question(s)
Severe epigastric pain	Does this patient have AAA?	What is causing the pain? If AAA, is it leaking?
Blunt abdominal trauma (FAST)	Is there free intraperitoneal fluid?	Is there solid organ injury? Is there a viscus rupture?
Painful leg	Is there an above-knee DVT?	What is causing the pain?
Painful hip	Is there an effusion?	Is there an infection?
Shock and chest pain	Is there a pericardial tamponade?	Is there a myocardial infarct?

AAA = abdominal aortic aneurysm; DVT = deep vein thrombosis; FAST = focused abdominal sonography in trauma.

The clinical question to be answered

Ideally, the question should have a **binary answer (yes/no)**. For example, 'Does the patient have an aortic aneurysm?' rather than 'What is causing this patient's abdominal pain?' Unlike formal ultrasound, emergency US uses a few, clearly defined views to answer binary questions very quickly. An understanding of this concept is absolutely fundamental to the safe interpretation of images.

Asking the wrong question is worse than useless. It is **dangerous** and fails to recognize the limitations of emergency US. For example, a negative FAST scan will lead to false reassurance if you fail to understand that it does not rule out solid organ injury.

Limitations of emergency US

Not all binary questions can be answered. US must be **capable** of answering the clinical question. For example, US is sensitive in the detection of hydronephrosis but poor at identifying ureteric stones. Therefore, in a patient with suspected ureteric colic, the right questions (those US can answer) are:

- Does this patient have abdominal aortic aneurysm (AAA) (as a differential diagnosis)?
- Does this patient have hydronephrosis (implying obstruction by a calculus)?
- Can I identify a calculus?

The wrong question:

- Can I **exclude** a calculus?

Operator and technical limitations

As discussed above, you are not a radiologist. Hence, some questions that experts can answer with US are beyond the reach of emergency sonographers. An echocardiographer using highly specialized equipment can identify pathology not visible to the emergency sonographer using a basic machine.

Furthermore, when you begin scanning you are not yet an emergency sonographer. The temptation to make clinical decisions based on scan results may be overwhelming for the beginner. However, all new diagnostic and therapeutic techniques require a programme of credentialing and ongoing maintenance of standards. Until the operator has achieved a minimum level of experience, great caution must be exercised in the performance and interpretation of emergency US scans for any new indication.

Will a scan change management in the emergency department?

There is little point performing examinations that are better performed by others unless there is a clear benefit to the patient or the department. For example, it is possible to identify many paediatric limb fractures on US. However, if one is also planning a diagnostic X-ray then US will cause the patient unnecessary distress.

Similarly, US identification of hydronephrosis matters little if the clinician requires CT to diagnose ureteric colic. However, the finding of hydronephrosis matters a great deal in a patient with acute renal failure as prompt decompression may prevent progression to dialysis.

Summary

→ Emergency US is rapid, safe, sensitive and allows ongoing resuscitation of the patient in the Emergency Department (ED).

→ It allows rapid (yes/no) answers to specific binary questions.

→ It is extremely dependent on operator and equipment limitations.

→ Like all ED investigations, it is indicated only if it will change management.

→ It is **not a substitute** for formal US by radiologists.

Chapter 2

How ultrasound works

Roslyn E Bell

What is ultrasound?

Ultrasound (US) uses high-frequency sound waves which are transmitted through the body from a transducer (probe). US waves are of much higher frequency than waves at the limit of human hearing; they usually range from 2 to 15 Megahertz (1 Hertz = 1 cycle/second), with higher frequencies (e.g. 7–12 MHz) used for more superficial scanning, and 3.5–5 MHz transducers most commonly used for abdominal scanning. As frequency increases, resolution improves but the ability to penetrate to deeper structures decreases (Fig. 2.1).

Types of US

There are several different modes of US, including A-mode used in scanning the eye, M-mode used in echocardiography, B-mode used in abdominal and musculoskeletal scanning, and Doppler imaging used when imaging flowing blood (in conjunction with B-mode).

In the A-mode, echoes are displayed on the screen in the form of a graph, with the x-axis representing time, and therefore depth, and the y-axis representing amplitude.

In the M mode, a sequence of repetitive A scans are recorded to show movement such as the movement of heart valves in echocardiography.

B-mode scanning is the type used in emergency department US. In this mode the US beam is swept through the patient's body, producing a two-dimensional (2D) scan plane. The tissues are represented on the screen in the form of a myriad of tiny white dots, which together form a 2D image.

Producing the image

The ultrasound pulses are produced within the transducer (probe) by passing an electromagnetic wave through a piezoelectric crystal causing it to vibrate. After each pulse has been produced the transducer switches to receiving mode. The transducer acts in the receiving mode for most of the time. The waves reflected back from the tissue boundaries cause the crystal to vibrate and produce an electrical signal. The probe's 'matching layer' improves energy transmission (Figure 2.2).

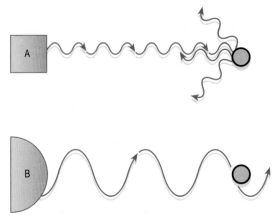

Fig. 2.1 *High-frequency sound waves (probe A) have better resolution and will be reflected by smaller objects compared to low-frequency waves (probe B).*

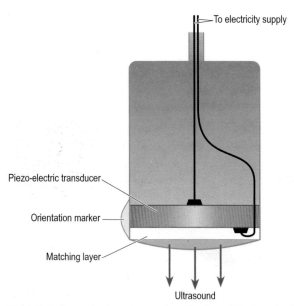

Fig. 2.2 *Probe and orientation marker. The 'matching layer', which is made of epoxy resin, improves energy transmission.*

Ultrasound waves travel at slightly different speeds through different tissues, and are reflected, absorbed or scattered at the boundaries between different media. When US waves hit these boundaries 'echoes' are sent back to the probe and are detected and analysed to form the image. The image on the screen is displayed as a series of dots, and the position of each of these dots depends on the time taken for the echo to return to the transducer. Echoes from deeper tissues take longer to return to the probe and are therefore positioned accordingly on the display. The brightness of each dot corresponds to the echo amplitude. Each ultrasound pulse from the transducer produces a series of dots, and many pulses are used to produce a cross-sectional image.

Sound energy travels through different media at different speeds. Approximate values are given in Table 2.1.

Each medium has different impedance to the passage of the sound wave, called its acoustic impedance. The greater the difference in acoustic impedance at a boundary, the greater the reflection of the sound wave.

It is therefore the varying properties and 'textures' of tissues that produce the different echoes, and consequently the differing 'echogenicities' of tissues seen on the image. Some examples (Figs 2.3 and 2.4):

Table 2.1 Ultrasound: speed through various media

Medium	Speed of sound (metres/sec)
Soft tissue	1570
Bone	3000
Water	1480
Fat	1450
Air	330

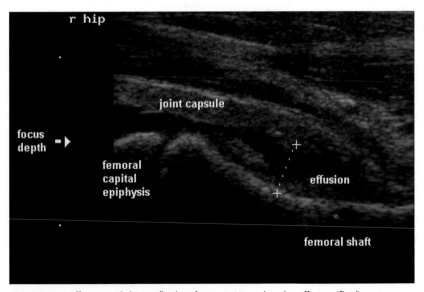

r hip

joint capsule

focus depth

femoral capital epiphysis

effusion

femoral shaft

Fig. 2.3 *Hip effusion with bone, fluid, soft tissue. Note that the effusion (fluid) appears black. A focus arrow is labelled at the side of the image.*

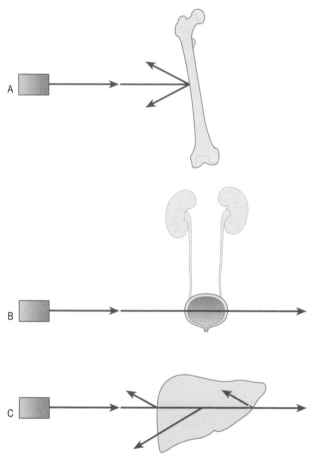

Fig. 2.4 Bone (A) is highly reflective and appears white. Fluid in the bladder (B) transmits sound and appears black. The liver (C), which reflects some sound and transmits the rest, appears grey.

- Bone cortex and calcified gallstones are highly reflective and appear white.
- Fluid (e.g. in bladder) transmits sound waves and appears black.
- Soft tissue (e.g. liver) is part-way between the two and appears grey.

Ultrasound gel is used between the probe and the patient as a 'coupling' agent because ultrasound waves require a transport medium and do not pass well through air.

The transducer

The most commonly used transducers (Fig. 2.5) in modern medical ultrasound are linear array and phased array, both of which have a row of small separate piezo-electric transducer (PZT) elements.

Linear array transducers produce a rectangular image, are generally of higher frequency—for example, 7–12 MHz—and are used to produce high-resolution images when scanning superficial and

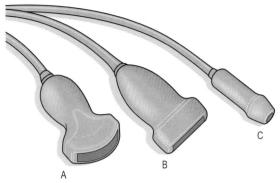

Fig. 2.5 *Transducers. (A) Low-frequency curved probe. (B) High-frequency linear array probe. (C) Phased-array microconvex probe.*

musculoskeletal structures. The PZT elements are activated electronically in sequence. Curvilinear transducers are essentially linear transducers constructed with a curve. They provide a wider field of view and are more suitable for deeper structures as the most superficial layers are distorted by the curved probe.

Phased array, or sector, transducers produce ultrasound beams by the PZT elements that are electronically steered by applying the voltage to the elements with small time differences. The beam is therefore swept through the tissues to produce a wide field of view image. These can be used in abdominal scanning and echocardiography, and are useful for areas that require a small 'footprint', for example, between ribs, as the transducer head is usually smaller than that of a curvilinear probe.

Orientation

It is important always to hold the probe in the correct orientation, as this will allow rapid identification of anatomy and the production of reliable and comparable images. On the image the patient's skin is at the top of the screen, and deeper structures towards the bottom of the screen.

When scanning longitudinally (sagittally), the patient's *head* should lie to the left of the screen and feet to the right. A longitudinal scan is shown in Figure 2.6.

When imaging in the transverse plane the patient's *right side* should lie to the left of the screen. A transverse scan is shown in Figure 2.7.

The probe is usually marked with a small light or other marker at one side, which should point to the patient's head for a longitudinal scan or the patient's right for a transverse scan (Fig. 2.2). Alternatively, by tapping a finger gently on one side of the probe the user can check image alignment.

The keyboard

The following are the important knobs (Fig. 2.8) used during a routine ED scan. There may be some variation in the labelling of these knobs on some makes of machine but these are the most commonly used.

Gain

Turning up the gain amplifies the signal from the returning echoes, making the

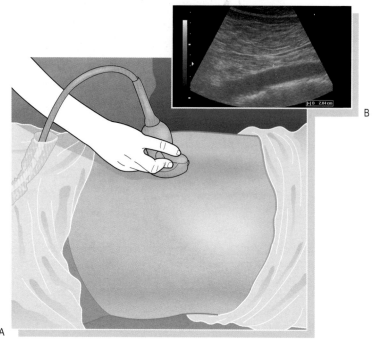

B

A

Fig. 2.6 *Longitudinal scan. (A) Probe orientation on body. (B) US image showing the upper aorta (in the lower part of the image); note that the blood-filled (i.e. fluid-filled) aorta is darker than the surrounding tissue.*

image more white and less dark. At the appropriate gain setting the image should be neither too bright nor too dark, and the distribution should be uniform from top to bottom of the image.

Time gain compensation
This is the set of slide bars on the keyboard that allow adjustment of gain at different levels of the image, for example, deeper layers may need increased gain.

Depth
This increases/decreases the depth of tissue visible; for example, depth is decreased to maximize the image of superficial structures and is increased to visualize deeper structures.

Focus/position
Arrow(s) at the side of the image (Fig. 2.3) designate the focal zone(s). They can be moved to sharpen the image at the level of interest.

Freeze
This button should be pressed to freeze the image prior to printing, or performing measurements.

Artefacts

An artefact is an image, or part of an image, that does not correspond to anatomy at that position in the patient. Artefacts can be useful in the interpretation of an image, or can obscure information. Examples of artefact include:

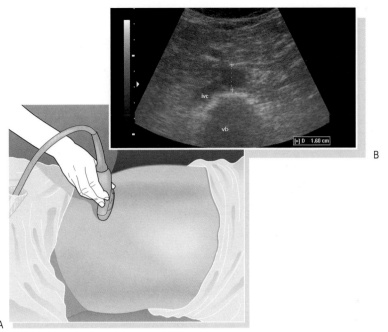

Fig. 2.7 Transverse scan. (A) Probe orientation on body. (B) A cross-section of the lower aorta is shown in the centre of this US image. ivc = inferior vena cava; vb = vertebral body.

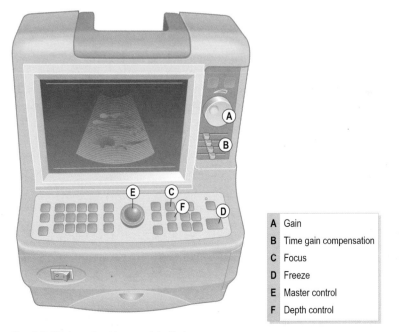

A	Gain
B	Time gain compensation
C	Focus
D	Freeze
E	Master control
F	Depth control

Fig. 2.8 Keyboard, with parts labelled.

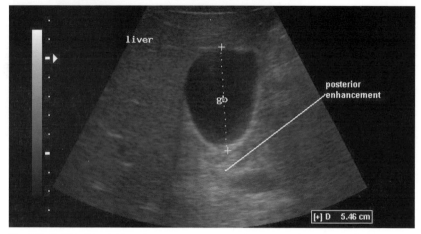

Fig. 2.9 Gallbladder (gb) and posterior acoustic enhancement (see section 'Acoustic enhancement and acoustic windows').

Acoustic enhancement and acoustic windows (Fig. 2.9)

Acoustic enhancement occurs when sound energy passes through a fluid-filled structure (e.g. urinary bladder, cysts, blood vessels). More sound energy passes through the tissues and returns to the probe (less attenuation), so tissues behind the fluid appear bright. Hence, the fluid acts as an 'acoustic window' for deeper structures. For example, in pelvic scans a full bladder acts as an acoustic window to help visualize deeper tissues.

Acoustic shadowing

This is the opposite of acoustic enhancement and occurs when sound energy hits a highly reflective structure (e.g. bone cortex or calculi) leaving little ultrasound energy to reach deeper structures. The tissues behind appear dark. This can be useful when scanning the gallbladder as gallstones can be recognized by their posterior 'comet tail' shadow (Fig. 2.10). However, shadowing can be problematic. For example, shadowing caused by ribs in the upper abdomen and chest can obscure deeper structures

(Fig. 2.11), and in older people leg veins can be obscured by calcified arteries.

Edge shadows

These are shadows cast by the curved walls of some rounded structures, such as gallbladder or blood vessel, due to strong reflection from the convex surface.

Mirror image (Fig. 2.12)

This is caused by reflection between a structure and a large curved interface. The time of the echo return is delayed and therefore the on-screen images are placed deeper than their actual location. A 'mirror image' of the structure appears on the other side of the interface, for example, mirror image of bladder in pelvis.

Reverberation (Fig. 2.13)

This appears as parallel, evenly spaced lines and is caused by multiple sound wave reflections between a structure and the probe or between two structures. The sound wave 'bounces' and returns to the probe more than once, producing an image with each reflection. This can occur if too little gel is used.

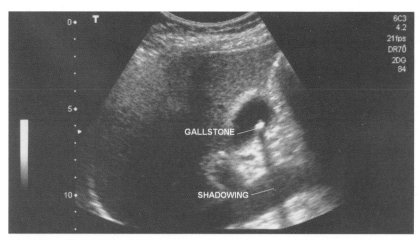

Fig. 2.10 Gallstone with posterior acoustic shadowing. *(See section 'Acoustic shadowing'.)*

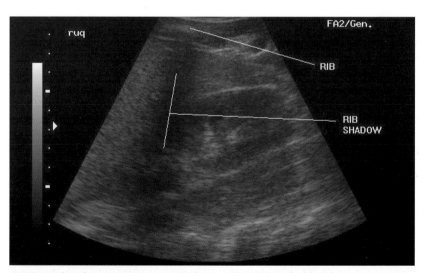

Fig. 2.11 Rib with posterior acoustic shadowing. The rib has shielded deeper structures from sound energy. The ability of acoustic shadowing to obscure deeper structures can be problematic. *(See section 'Acoustic shadowing'.)*

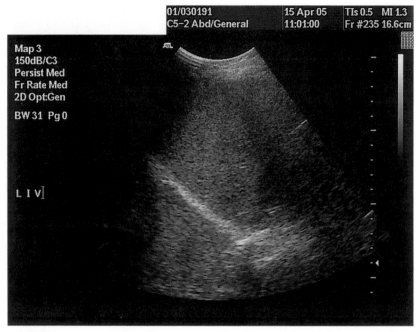

Fig. 2.12 *A mirror image of the liver is identified on the cranial side of the diaphragm.*

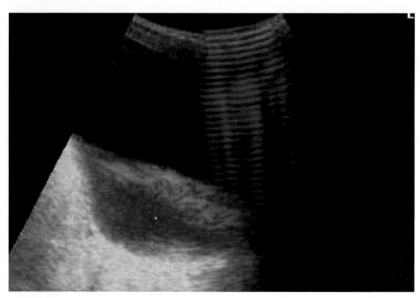

Fig. 2.13 *Transverse scan of bladder demonstrating reverberation artefact on right of image.*

Handy hints

✔ When starting work with a new US machine familiarize yourself with the keyboard layout and functions as there is considerable variation between products.

✔ Orientate the probe prior to each scan to avoid confusion:

   ✔ longitudinal scan: patient's *head* lies to the left of the screen;

   ✔ transverse scan: patient's *right side* lies to the left of the screen.

✔ Use more gel if in doubt.

✔ If you are having difficulty obtaining or interpreting an image consider the three Ps:

   ✔ Probe: orientation, gain, gel;

   ✔ Patient: genuine pathology, acoustic shadowing (e.g. ribs), bowel gas (US passes poorly through air), obesity;

   ✔ Physics: mirror artefact, reverberation.

Summary

→ B-mode US is the type used in the emergency department.

→ Higher frequency linear probes are used for more superficial scans and lower frequency curvilinear or phased array transducers for greater depth.

→ US gel is used between the probe and the patient.

→ Different tissues have different appearances, for example, bone cortex appears white and water appears black.

→ On the image the patient's skin is at the top of the screen, and deeper structures towards the bottom of the screen.

→ Longitudinal scan: patient's *head* lies to the left of the screen.

→ Transverse scan: patient's *right side* lies to the left of the screen.

→ Image artefact can be confusing or obscure anatomy, but can be helpful in some cases.

Chapter 3

Abdominal aorta

Justin Bowra

The question: is there an abdominal aortic aneurysm?

The abdominal aorta passes from the diaphragm (surface anatomy: xiphoid process) distally through the retroperitoneum until its bifurcation into the common iliac arteries (approximately at the level of the fourth lumbar vertebra, surface anatomy: approximately at umbilicus) (Fig. 3.1). In adults its normal anteroposterior (AP) diameter is less than 2 cm. A dilatation of the aorta 3 cm or more (i.e. 1.5× normal) is known as an abdominal aortic aneurysm (AAA) and may be fusiform or saccular. Most aneurysms occur below the renal arteries.

Abdominal aorta AP diameter (Fig. 3.2):

- <2 cm normal
- 2–3 cm dilated but not aneurysmal
- >3 cm aneurysm

The larger the aneurysm the faster it dilates (LaPlace's law) and the greater its risk of rupture. The risk of rupture is small if the diameter is less than 5 cm. The elective operative mortality is approximately 5%. However, the mortality of ruptured AAA is 50% *provided the patient reaches the operating theatre (OT).*

Why use ultrasound?

Physical examination is unreliable in making the diagnosis. Alternative imaging techniques (such as CT) take time to organize and require the transfer of an unstable patient out of the Emergency Department (ED). Bedside US is rapid, safe, sensitive (97–100%) and allows ongoing resuscitation of the patient in the ED. Doppler imaging adds little and is not required.

Clinical picture

The clinical picture and its variability will be familiar to the experienced clinician.

- *The patient*: usually male (10 × more common) and older than 50 years.
- *Pain*: usually severe abdominal pain, which may radiate to the back.
- *Shock*: not always present (e.g. contained rupture).
- *Abdominal mass*: above the umbilicus. Its absence does not rule out AAA.
- *Distal pulses*: usually normal.
- *Other presentations*: rare, for example mass effect (such as bowel obstruction), torrential gastrointestinal bleeding from aortoenteric fistula.

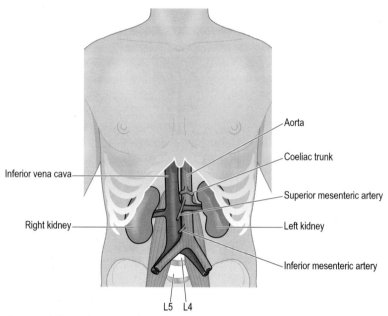

Fig. 3.1 *Abdominal aorta and its relations.*

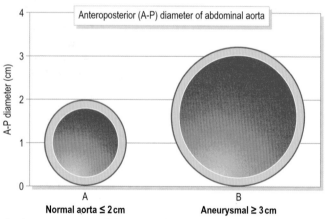

Fig. 3.2 *Comparison of diameters of normal and aneurysmal aorta.*

Broad differential diagnosis: for example, perforated viscus, peptic ulcer disease, acute coronary syndromes.

 If in doubt, assume that the patient has AAA until proven otherwise.

Before you scan

- Move the patient to the resuscitation area.
- Address ABCs. (N.B. Aggressive fluid resuscitation of AAA may be detrimental. The optimum systolic BP is probably 90–100 mmHg.)
- Get help: the doctor performing the scan should not also be resuscitating the patient.

 ED investigations (including US) and treatment must not delay urgent transfer of a shocked patient with suspected AAA to operation.

The technique and views

Patient's position
- Dictated by clinical picture;
- Supine is most practical.

Probe and scanner settings
- Curved probe: standard 2.5–3.5 MHz is ideal;
- Standard B-mode setting;
- Focus depth 10 cm;
- Depth setting 15–20 cm.

Probe placement and landmarks
1. Start just below xiphisternum. Transverse position with probe marker to patient's right (Fig. 3.3).
2. Identify landmarks: vertebral body (VB, confirm bone's acoustic shadow) directly behind aorta, liver anterior and to the right, bowel (Fig. 3.4).
3. It is essential to identify and differentiate the *two* major vessels: inferior vena cava (IVC) and aorta (Table 3.1). The IVC is parallel and to the right and may be misidentified as the aorta, particularly in longitudinal section. Transmitted pulsation in the IVC can be misleading.
4. Alter the depth setting, focus depth and gain to obtain the best image.
5. Measure AP diameter, save and print image.
6. Maintain the transverse position and sweep distally until bifurcation (Fig. 3.5): measure diameter, save and print image.
7. Move the probe to longitudinal position and scan. Attempt to obtain a view of the aorta with origin of coeliac trunk or superior mesenteric artery (SMA) (Fig. 3.6).

Table 3.1 Identification of the major blood vessels

Inferior vena cava	Aorta
To the anatomical right (*left* on screen)	To the left
Compressible (unless distal obstruction e.g. massive PE)	Non-compressible
Thinner walls	Thick walled, calcified
Oval cross section	Round cross section Smaller unless AAA

AAA = abdominal aortic aneurysm; PE = pulmonary embolism.

19

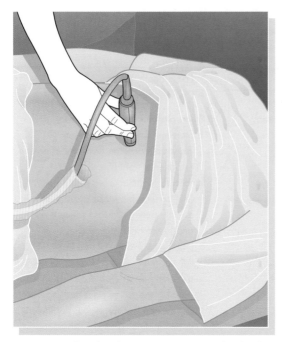

Fig. 3.3 Initial probe placement: transverse subxiphoid, probe directed posteriorly and probe marker to patient's right.

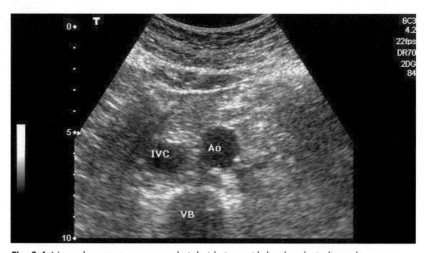

Fig. 3.4 Normal aorta, transverse subxiphoid view with landmarks indicated.

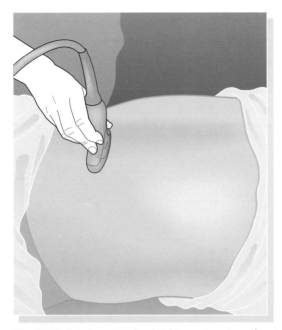

Fig. 3.5 *Probe placement for distal transverse view of aorta.*

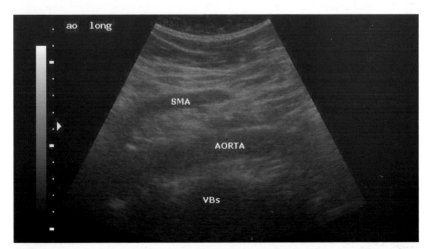

Fig. 3.6 *Normal aorta longitudinal view (below) with origin of superior mesenteric artery (above).*

Essential views

To rule out AAA, the aorta should be visualized in its entirety and a minimum of three hard copy images should be obtained:

- upper transverse section (Fig. 3.4)
- lower transverse section
- longitudinal section (ideally with origin of coeliac trunk or SMA) (Fig. 3.6).

All three views must include measurement of diameter.

 You have not ruled out AAA unless you can visualize the entire length of the aorta.

Positives and negatives

- Normal aorta <2 cm diameter (Fig. 3.4)
- Aneurysm >3 cm (Figs 3.7, 3.8, 3.10)
- Inadequate image (Fig. 3.11).

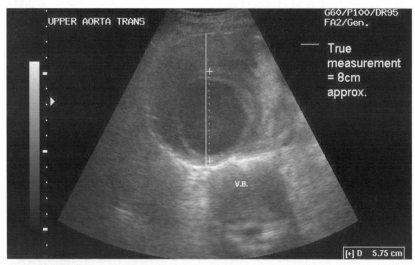

Fig. 3.7 *Abdominal aortic aneurysm (AAA) with mural thrombus, transverse section. Two anteroposterior (AP) measurements: the measurement between 'inner walls' underestimates the AP diameter. V.B. = vertebral body.*

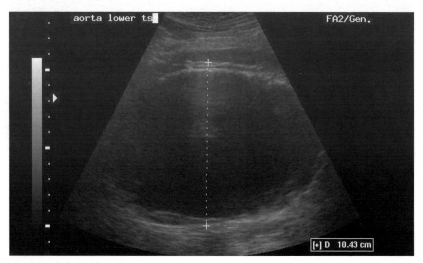

Fig. 3.8 *Abdominal aortic aneurysm (AAA) with correct (perpendicular) estimation of diameter.*

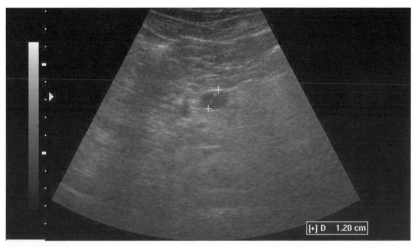

Fig. 3.9 Abdominal aorta, incorrect (angled) estimation of diameter. Inadequate image, focus arrow set correctly but depth and gain settings are suboptimal.

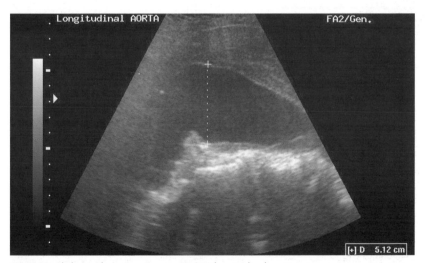

Fig. 3.10 Abdominal aortic aneurysm (AAA) longitudinal section.

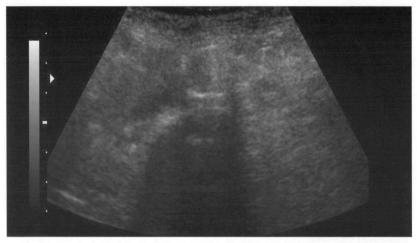

Fig. 3.11 *Uninterpretable US image. Calcified oval structure is probably the aorta, but is not well demonstrated. Gain and depth should be decreased.*

Handy hints

✔ Despite a skilled operator, sometimes bowel gas may render an image inadequate. If bowel gas is in the way, continue direct pressure with the probe on the abdominal wall (if pain permits) to displace the bowel. Altering the angle of the transducer may also help.

✔ Obese patients may be very difficult. Increasing the image depth and altering the focus may help.

✔ Measure diameter between the *outer* margins of each wall, not inner: this may overestimate the diameter but will avoid false negatives due to mural thrombus (Fig. 3.7).

✔ The aorta may be ectatic and this will make measurement of diameter difficult. However, attempt to measure the diameter perpendicularly (Fig. 3.8); avoid taking a slice at an angle (Fig. 3.9) as this will overestimate the diameter.

✔ If on the first or second view you demonstrate AAA in an unstable patient your priority is to transfer the patient to an operating theatre. Further views are not needed and waste time.

What US can tell you

• Is there an aneurysm (AAA)? US can detect AAA in at least 97% of cases, depending on operator and patient factors (e.g. obesity).

What US can't tell you

• Is the aneurysm leaking? US is insensitive in detection of retroperitoneal blood. If you detect AAA in a shocked patient, *assume* that it has ruptured or is leaking.

• Other causes of the pain. The differential diagnosis of severe epigastric pain in an unstable patient is broad. None of these differentials can be diagnosed or ruled out accurately by emergency US.

Now what?

- Unstable patient and AAA: notify surgical team immediately. The patient must be transferred immediately to the OT for AAA repair.
- Unstable patient, unable to rule out AAA: this is a complex situation. Ongoing resuscitation, urgent surgical review and decision to proceed to OT (or further imaging such as CT) must be based on clinical likelihood of AAA.
- AAA ruled out by US: look for other cause of presentation (see above).
- Stable patient and AAA (or unable to rule out AAA): discuss with vascular surgeons. Patient requires further assessment and imaging (e.g. CT) to assess extent, renal artery involvement etc.

Summary

→ Bedside US for suspected AAA is rapid, safe, sensitive and allows ongoing resuscitation of the patient in the ED.

→ However, US and other ED investigations *must not delay* urgent transfer of a shocked patient with suspected AAA to the OT.

→ If in doubt, assume that the patient has AAA.

→ If you detect AAA in a shocked patient, *assume* that it has ruptured or is leaking.

→ You have not ruled out AAA unless you can visualize the entire length of the aorta.

→ To rule out AAA, a minimum of three views should be obtained: upper and lower transverse sections and a longitudinal section. All three views must include measurement of diameter.

Chapter 4

Focused assessment with sonography in trauma (FAST)

Russell McLaughlin

The question: is there free fluid?

Focused assessment with sonography in trauma (FAST) is a means of detecting free intraperitoneal fluid in the traumatized abdomen. Using ATLS® (Advanced Trauma Life Support) principles, the FAST scan is used as an adjunct to the primary survey assessment of circulation. It relies on the principle that, in the supine patient, free fluid (FF) such as blood collects in certain anatomical sites.

In the thorax, FF may be found in one of two potential spaces: the pericardium and pleural space. Pericardial blood, particularly if it collects rapidly, will progressively impair right ventricular diastolic filling until tamponade occurs. In a supine patient with a haemothorax, blood initially collects at the posterior lung bases. Like pericardial tamponade, massive haemothorax is a life-threatening condition that requires immediate drainage. The author advises that the lung bases should routinely be included in FAST views.

In the supine abdomen, the most dependent potential spaces are scanned by FAST. Morison's pouch is found between the liver and right kidney. FF will collect here first. The lienorenal interface is the analogous potential space between the spleen and left kidney. Fluid on the left side will collect here or above the spleen (subphrenic fluid). In the pelvis, FF will collect in the pouch of Douglas (rectovesical pouch in the male) behind the bladder.

Why use ultrasound?

- Traumatic cardiac tamponade and massive haemothorax may be rapidly fatal if not detected and treated in the Emergency Department (ED).
- Physical examination is unreliable for detection of cardiac tamponade in the ED setting.
- US can be used to guide emergent pericardiocentesis and intercostal catheter placement.

- Physical examination is only 50–60% sensitive for detecting abdominal injury following blunt trauma.
- FAST is easy to learn. Reliable and repeatable results can be achieved after as little as 10 proctored scans.
- FAST is non-invasive, rapid, repeatable and can be performed at the bedside.
- FAST has supplanted diagnostic peritoneal lavage (DPL) as a reliable and non-invasive means of detecting abdominal FF in trauma patients.
- FAST is up to 90% sensitive and up to 99% specific for traumatic haemoperitoneum. (See *Cautions and contraindications*, below.)

Clinical picture

- *The patient.* The patient will have suffered a form of trauma in which cardiac tamponade, intrathoracic or intraperitoneal bleeding is a possibility.

Cautions and contraindications

- The only absolute contraindications to performing a FAST scan are the presence of a more pressing problem (such as airway obstruction) or a clear indication for emergency laparotomy (in which case FAST is not indicated).
- FAST is indicated only if it will affect patient management. For example, in the stable patient with blunt abdominal trauma, a negative FAST gives no information about solid organs or hollow viscus injury. Such patients may require other imaging such as CT.

- *Children.* FAST can be performed in children but CT scanning remains the investigation of choice in paediatric abdominal trauma. The threshold for operative intervention in paediatric blunt abdominal trauma is higher than for adults.
- *Timing.* A very early scan may be falsely negative as sufficient intra-abdominal blood may not have collected in the dependent areas. Furthermore, occasionally a late scan may be falsely negative as clotted blood is of similar echogenicity to liver and may not be easily identified in Morison's pouch.
- *Operator.* The accuracy of FAST is operator-dependent and the inexperienced scanner should be particularly wary of ruling out FF.

 Urgent surgical consultation is mandatory in the unstable trauma patient suspected of having intra-abdominal injury.

 FAST is indicated only if it will affect patient management.

 FAST is not indicated in patients with a clear indication for immediate laparotomy, for example, penetrating injury in an unstable patient.

Before you scan

- Move the patient to the resuscitation area and assemble trauma team.
- Primary survey and resuscitation according to ATLS principles.
- The doctor performing the scan should not also be resuscitating the patient.

Technique and views

Patient's position

The patient should be in the supine position with arms abducted slightly or above the head to allow visualization of Morison's pouch and the spleen. Alternatively, the patient may be asked to fold their arms across their chest. This manoeuvre will be determined by consciousness level of the patient and the presence of any upper extremity injury.

Probe and scanner settings

A low-frequency (4–7 MHz) probe should be used with the focus depth and depth set according to the patient's body habitus and the initial image obtained.

The 5 views (Fig. 4.1)

1. *Pericardium*. The most common view used in this situation is the subxiphoid view. The probe is laid almost flat on the patient's epigastrium and angled towards the head. Advance the probe toward the xiphisternum. Apply enough pressure to allow the probe to indent the epigastrium, thus placing the probe deeper than the xiphisternum and costal margin (Fig. 4.2). Then sweep the probe in a left-to-right axis until the pulsation of the myocardium is visualized. The view obtained utilizes the liver as an acoustic window (see Ch. 2) and should demonstrate the four chambers of the heart (Fig. 4.3). Pericardial fluid appears as a black stripe (Fig. 4.4). In true cardiac tamponade the right ventricle will collapse during diastole. However, this can be difficult to assess for the non-echocardiographer, so clinical likelihood of tamponade must be taken into consideration when acting on a positive scan. In some patients, particularly the obese, it may be difficult to obtain clear subxiphoid images. An alternative method in these patients is the left longitudinal parasternal view (Fig. 4.5).

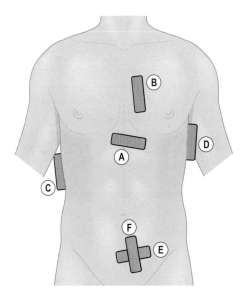

A	Subxiphoid
B	Left longitudinal parasternal
C	Morison's pouch
D	Lienorenal
E	Pelvis transverse
F	Pelvis sagittal

Fig. 4.1 *Windows used for the FAST examination.*

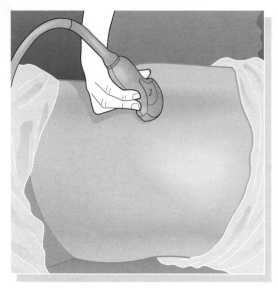

Fig. 4.2 *Probe in subxiphoid pericardial position.*

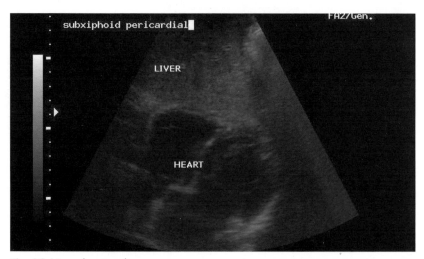

Fig. 4.3 *Normal pericardium.*

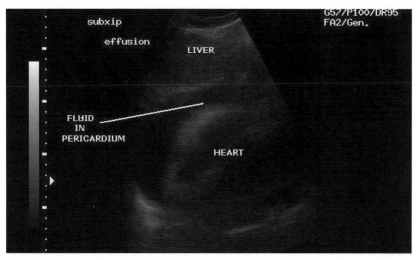

Fig. 4.4 *Pericardial fluid.*

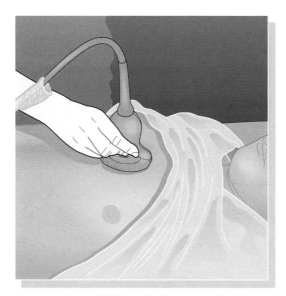

Fig. 4.5 *Probe in left longitudinal parasternal position.*

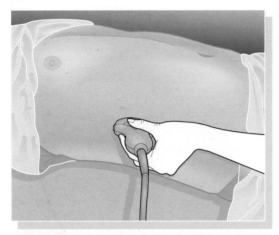

Fig. 4.6 Probe in Morison's pouch position.

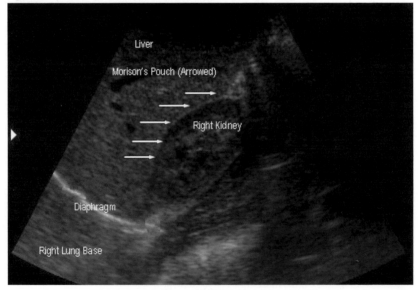

Fig. 4.7 Normal Morison's pouch.

2. *Morison's pouch and right lung base.*
   Probe parallel and between the ribs
   where the costal margin meets the mid-
   axillary line on the right of the patient
   (Fig. 4.6). The view obtained utilizes
   the liver as an acoustic window and
   should demonstrate right kidney, liver,
   diaphragm (highly echogenic) and
   right lung base for pneumo/
   haemothorax (Fig. 4.7). Sweep

the probe anteroposteriorly and
alter the probe angle until you obtain
a clear view of Morison's Pouch. FF
will appear as a black stripe in
Morison's pouch (Fig. 4.8). Ask the
patient to take a deep breath if
possible, particularly if rib shadows
obscure the area of interest: a clearer
view of the liver and Morison's pouch
is often obtained with this method.

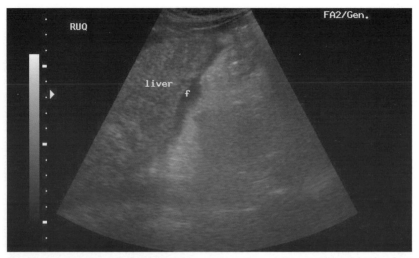

Fig. 4.8 *Free fluid (f) in Morison's pouch.*

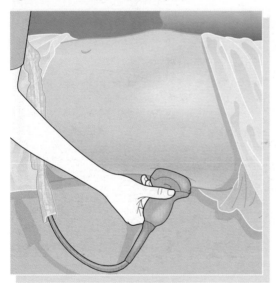

Fig. 4.9 *Probe in lienorenal position.*

3. *Lienorenal interface and left lung base.*
   Probe is angled on the left side as if
   looking for Morison's pouch but higher
   (ribs 9–11) and more posteriorly, in the
   posterior axillary line (Fig. 4.9). The
   spleen may be higher than expected
   and is more difficult to visualize than
   the liver. In a co-operative patient, a

deep breath may help. Sweep the
probe and alter its angle as above,
until you obtain a clear view of left
kidney, spleen, diaphragm and left
lung base (Fig. 4.10) FF will appear as
a black stripe in the lienorenal interface
(Fig. 4.11) or between the spleen and
the diaphragm (subphrenic FF).

33

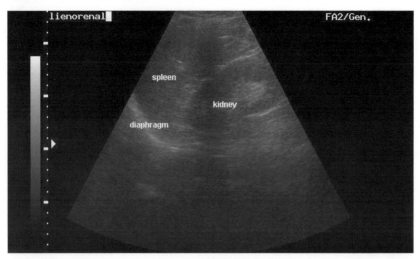

Fig. 4.10 *Normal lienorenal interface, landmarks labelled.*

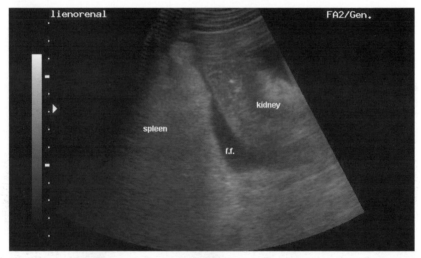

Fig. 4.11 *Free fluid (f.f.) in the lienorenal interface.*

4. *Pelvis: sagittal.* For both pelvic views the fluid-filled bladder is utilized as an acoustic window. It is therefore important that the patient has a full bladder during this part of the examination. Ideally scan before catheterizing the patient. Otherwise, depending on urgency, clamp the indwelling catheter and allow the bladder to fill or fill the bladder with normal saline via the catheter. To obtain the sagittal view, place the probe in the midline just above the pubis and angle it caudally at 45° into the pelvis (Fig. 4.12). The view obtained should demonstrate a coronal section of the bladder and pelvic organs (Fig. 4.13). FF will be around the bladder or behind it (pouch of Douglas) (Fig. 4.14).

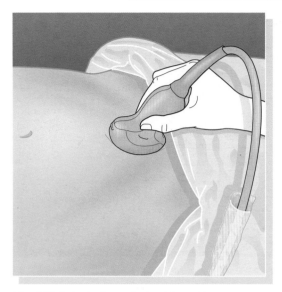

Fig. 4.12 *Probe in the sagittal pelvis position.*

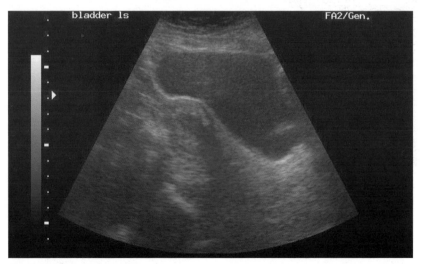

Fig. 4.13 *Sagittal view pelvis.*

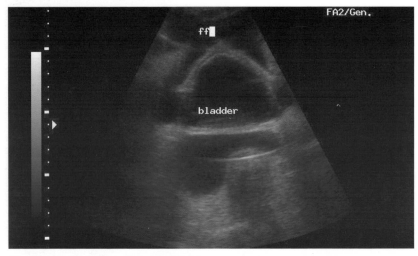

Fig. 4.14 *Free fluid (ff) in the sagittal pelvis.*

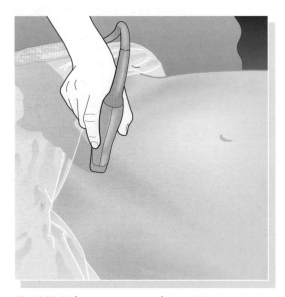

Fig. 4.15 *Probe in transverse pelvis position.*

5. *Pelvis: transverse.* This view is obtained by rotating the probe through 90° from the sagittal position while maintaining contact with the abdominal wall (Fig. 4.15). Angle the probe into the pelvis, identify the bladder in transverse section and sweep the probe to visualize the pouch of Douglas and pelvic organs as above (Fig. 4.16).

6. *Extra views.* Some authors recommend paracolic views. These probably do not add to the sensitivity of FAST and are not routine.

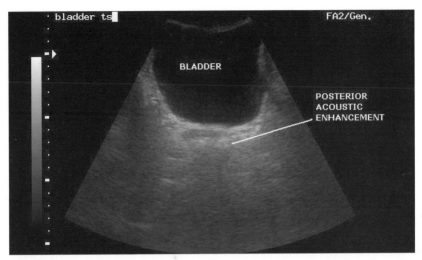

Fig. 4.16 *Transverse view pelvis.*

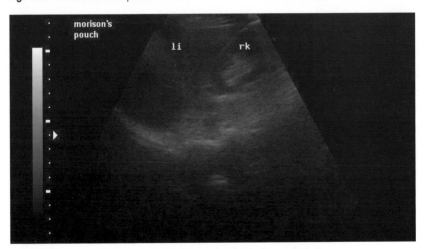

Fig. 4.17 *Morison's pouch: inadequate view. li = liver; rk = right kidney.*

Essential views

To rule out FF, a minimum of five hard-copy images should be obtained:

- pericardium
- Morison's pouch
- lienorenal interface
- pelvic sagittal
- pelvic transverse.

Positives and negatives

- Pericardium, no fluid (Fig. 4.3)
- Pericardial fluid (Fig. 4.4)
- Morison's pouch, no free fluid (Fig. 4.7)
- Morison's pouch, free fluid (Fig. 4.8)
- Morison's pouch, inadequate image (Fig. 4.17)
- Lienorenal interface, no free fluid (Fig. 4.10)

- Lienorenal interface, free fluid (Fig. 4.11)
- Transverse pelvis, no free fluid (Fig 4.16)
- Sagittal pelvis, free fluid (Fig. 4.13).

Handy hints

✔ Left longitudinal parasternal position provides an alternative view of the pericardium.

✔ The lienorenal interface is more posterior and more cranial than you think!

✔ Scan through the respiratory cycle to minimize the effects of rib shadowing.

✔ If available, a probe with a particularly small footprint can scan between ribs.

✔ If you still find it difficult to obtain clear views of Morison's pouch or the lienorenal space, slide the probe proximally until you view the highly echogenic diaphragm. Use this as the landmark to identify the adjacent pleural space and liver/spleen.

✔ Sometimes only subdiaphragmatic free fluid (FF) will be seen (particularly on the left), so scan between the liver/ spleen and diaphragm.

✔ Beware false-negative scans. In the presence of small amounts of FF, a single view of Morison's pouch or lienorenal interface may be falsely negative. Hence, scan through a number of planes to rule out FF. If you still suspect FF, consider serial scans or other investigation.

✔ Similarly, scan any positive findings of FF through a number of planes and observe for peristalsis, pulsation and displacement with respiration. This allows FF to be differentiated from false positives due to fluid-filled structures such as inferior vena cava, gall bladder and intraluminal bowel fluid.

✔ Other causes of false-positive scans include:
  ✔ fat (e.g. pericardial fat pad);
  ✔ ascites;
  ✔ mirror artefact (see below).

✔ Fluid in the bladder is required to visualize the pelvis.

✔ If FF in the pelvis cannot be distinguished from mirror artefact (see Ch. 2) scan the pelvis through a number of planes: only FF should persist. Alternatively, the bladder can be partially emptied. Mirror artefact 'shrinks' with the emptying bladder while FF remains constant.

✔ Repeat the scan, particularly if a stable patient becomes unstable.

✔ If, on the first or second view, you demonstrate FF in an unstable patient, further views are not needed and waste time.

What FAST can tell you

FAST can determine the presence of the following:

- free intraperitoneal fluid
- pericardial fluid
- pleural fluid.

What FAST can't tell you

FAST cannot determine the following:

- source of free fluid
- nature of free fluid, for example, blood versus ascites
- presence of solid organ or hollow viscus injury
- presence of retroperitoneal injury.

Now what?

 Urgent surgical consultation is mandatory in the unstable trauma patient with suspected intra-abdominal injury.

 FAST is not indicated in patients with a clear indication for immediate laparotomy, for example, penetrating injury in an unstable patient.

Abdominal injury without clear indication for immediate laparotomy:

- Unstable patient and pericardial fluid: suspect cardiac tamponade. Prepare for emergent pericardiocentesis.
- Unstable patient and pleural FF: suspect massive haemothorax. Emergent intercostal catheter drainage.
- Unstable patient and intra-abdominal FF: immediate transfer to theatre for laparotomy.

- Unstable patient, inadequate or negative scan: ongoing resuscitation, clinical reassessment for other cause of instability, consider other investigation (e.g. CT, DPL) or exploratory laparotomy. While still in ED, frequent re-scanning for subsequent fluid accumulation.
- Stable patient and negative scan: although FF is excluded, assess patient for solid organ and hollow viscus injury as well as extra-abdominal injuries.
- Stable patient and positive scan: abdominal CT.

Summary

→ FAST is useful when assessing the traumatized abdomen.
→ FAST is indicated only if it will affect patient management.
→ It does not replace sound clinical judgement.
→ It must be used in conjunction with ATLS principles.

Chapter 5

Deep vein thrombosis

Niall Collum, Charles Martyn

The question: is there a deep vein thrombosis?

Deep vein thrombosis (DVT) is the 3rd most common cardiovascular disease in the USA, after acute coronary syndrome and stroke, affecting 2 million individuals per annum. The annual incidence of DVT in the UK is 0.5–1 per 1000 adults: i.e. up to 60 000 cases per annum. Pulmonary embolism (PE) is recognized as the cause of death in approximately 8000 people per annum in the UK, and 90% of PE have DVT as the source. In reality, the incidence of both PE and DVT is probably much higher due to significant underdiagnosis.

Many patients will present themselves, or be referred by their GP to the Emergency Department (ED) for investigation with a painful or swollen leg. Clinical examination for DVT is unreliable, and further investigation is often required.

It is crucial that the diagnosis of DVT be made quickly and accurately, allowing treatment to be instituted at an early stage.

Why use compression ultrasound?

Compression ultrasound (compression US) has become the diagnostic modality of choice by radiologists for symptomatic DVT with both sensitivity and specificity of 98–100% reported for proximal DVT. In addition, compression US in the ED has been shown to reduce significantly the time to diagnosis for this group of patients.

Three-point compression US is a simplification of standard compression US that is easily learned, rapid to perform, and has been shown to be highly accurate in the diagnosis of proximal DVT. Sensitivity of 93–100% and specificity of 97–100% for proximal DVT is reported. Benefits include diagnosis at point of care, streamlined patient flow and decreased pressure on radiology services.

A limitation of three-point compression US is missed isolated *below-knee* DVT. However, many clinicians consider that in patients with isolated below-knee DVT the drawbacks of anticoagulation (risk of complications, cost and inconvenience) may exceed the benefits.

Table 5.1 Wells' criteria: a clinical risk assessment tool

Clinical parameter score	Score
Active cancer (treatment ongoing, or within 6 months or palliative)	+1
Paralysis or recent plaster immobilization of the lower extremities	+1
Recently bedridden for >3 days or major surgery <4 weeks	+1
Localized tenderness along the distribution of the deep venous system	+1
Entire leg swelling	+1
Calf swelling >3 cm compared to the asymptomatic leg	+1
Pitting oedema (greater in the symptomatic leg)	+1
Previous DVT documented	+1
Collateral superficial veins (non-varicose)	+1
Alternative diagnosis (as likely or > that of DVT)	−2

Total of above score

High probability of DVT	2 or more
Low probability	less than 2

DVT = deep vein thrombosis.

In DVT the major health risks are propagation and/or embolization. The risk of embolization in a patient who may have *below-knee* DVT, but with no evidence of proximal DVT on compression US, is between 0.7% and 1.1%. However, the risk of propagation of below-knee DVT is quoted as ranging from 2% to 36%. Patients therefore who have normal three-point compression testing, but who are at high risk for DVT as defined by a validated clinical assessment tool, should have a repeat scan at 1 week. Local treatment protocols should be followed as regards the need for anticoagulation during this period.

An example of a clinical risk assessment tool (Wells' criteria) is given in Table 5.1.

Anatomy (Fig. 5.1)

- The popliteal vein begins as the confluence of the calf veins behind the knee. It lies superficial to the popliteal artery in the popliteal fossa, and ascends to the adductor canal where it becomes the femoral vein (also known as the superficial femoral vein).
- The femoral vein is found anteromedially in the thigh: initially deep to the femoral artery, coming to lie more medially as it ascends. The profunda femoris vein joins the femoral vein approximately 4 cm below the inguinal ligament, becoming the common femoral vein.
- The long saphenous vein joins just proximal to the common femoral vein. The common femoral vein becomes the external iliac vein as it passes superiorly, under the inguinal ligament.

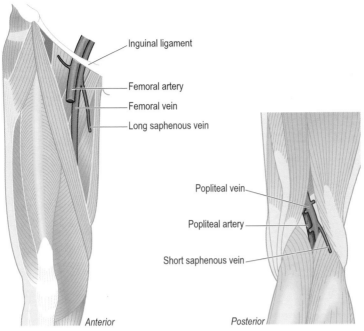

Fig. 5.1 *Relations of the femoral and popliteal veins.*

Clinical picture

This is often unreliable. If in doubt, assume that the patient has DVT until proven otherwise.

- The history: classically, a history of atraumatic calf or thigh pain and swelling, with recognized risk factors such as immobilization, recent surgery, smoking and active cancer.
- The examination: classically leg swelling, calf tenderness along the distribution of the deep veins, pitting oedema in the symptomatic leg and absence of a likely alternative diagnosis.
- Associated symptoms/signs of pulmonary embolus (PE) may be present: collapse; tachycardia; tachypnoea; hypotension; short of breath; pleuritic chest pain.

- Broad differential diagnosis: for example, symptomatic Baker's cyst, cellulitis, superficial thrombophlebitis, soft-tissue injury, lymphadenopathy.

 If in doubt, assume that the patient has DVT until proven otherwise.

Before you scan

- Ensure that the area to be used is private
- Darkened room
- Ensure that the patient is comfortable
- Have an adequate supply of ultrasound gel.

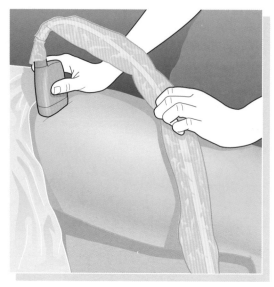

Fig. 5.2 *Initial patient position (supine) with probe at groin.*

The technique and views

Patient's position

Groin to adductor canal (Fig. 5.2)

- Supine, with acoustic jelly along the course of the femoral vein
- Leg abducted to 10–15°, slight external rotation.

Popliteal segment (Fig. 5.3)

- Partial decubitus, affected leg uppermost
- Knee flexed to 25–30° (removes tension on popliteal fascia and vein).

Probe and scanner settings

- Standard B-mode settings
- Linear transducer, high-frequency (5.0–7.5 MHz)
- Depth setting 3–4 cm
- Focus depth 3 cm.

Probe placement and landmarks

- Hold the probe in transverse position throughout, with the probe marker to the patient's right (Fig. 5.2). (If trying to compress veins in the longitudinal position, the probe may 'slip off' and give a false impression of compression.)
- Start in groin just below the midpoint of the inguinal ligament. Rest the probe lightly on the skin, identifying the 'Mickey Mouse' sign (Fig. 5.4):
  - Femoral artery (thick-walled) seen pulsating lateral to femoral vein
  - Saphenofemoral venous confluence: thinner-walled, transmitted pulsation only.

Gentle compression will appose the anterior and posterior walls of normal veins; arteries are relatively incompressible.

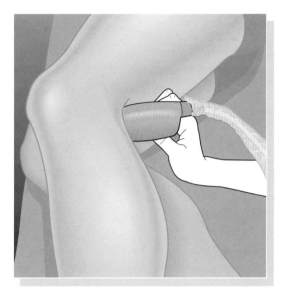

Fig. 5.3 Next patient position (partial decubitus) with probe in popliteal fossa.

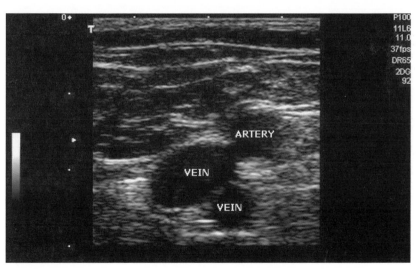

Fig. 5.4 Normal saphenofemoral confluence, no compression.

- Place the probe in the optimum position for saphenofemoral confluence. Record and print copies of two views: one without compression, one with compression, apposing the vein walls (Figs 5.4 and 5.5).

- Follow the femoral vein distally compressing and releasing, ideally until the entire length has been visualized to the adductor hiatus (see *Handy hints*, below). Record and print two views (Figs 5.6 and 5.7).

45

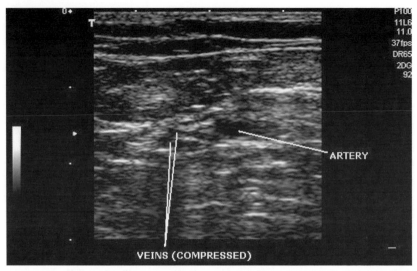

Fig. 5.5 *Normal saphenofemoral confluence, compression.*

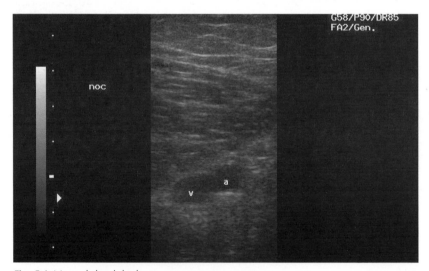

Fig. 5.6 *Normal distal thigh; no compression. v = vein; a = artery.*

- Re-position the patient as described above, to evaluate the popliteal segment.
- With the probe in the popliteal fossa, identify the popliteal vein lying superficially, with the artery pulsating deeply to this.

- Follow the popliteal vein superiorly to the adductor hiatus and inferiorly to the confluence into the calf veins, compressing and releasing. Record and print two views (Figs 5.8 and 5.9).

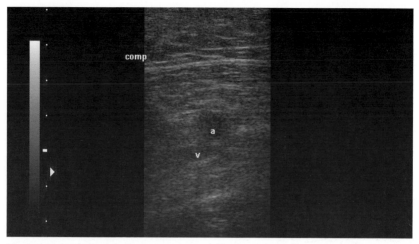

Fig. 5.7 *Normal distal thigh, compression. v = vein; a = artery.*

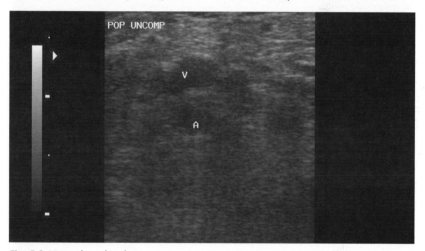

Fig. 5.8 *Normal popliteal, no compression. V = vein; A = artery.*

If at any point the vein is seen to have echogenic material within the lumen, and/or is found to be incompressible, then the patient has a DVT at this site. The examination can be terminated at this point (Fig. 5.10).

Essential views

A minimum of six views must be obtained:

- saphenofemoral confluence with and without compression
- distal femoral vein with and without compression
- popliteal vein with and without compression.

 All views should be clearly labelled with anatomical site, whether compression applied, and artery and veins identified.

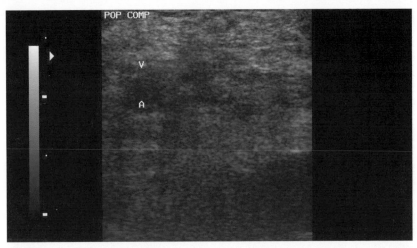

Fig. 5.9 Normal popliteal, compression. V = vein; A = artery.

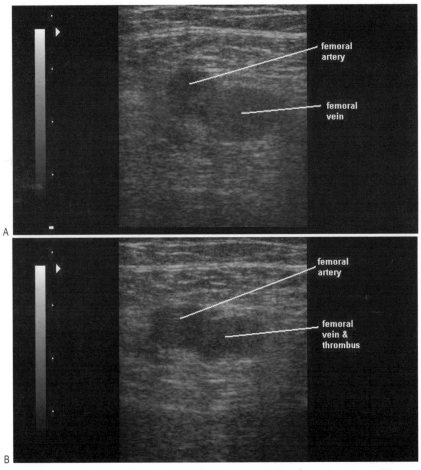

Fig. 5.10 Deep vein thrombosis (DVT) with compression (A) and no compression (B).

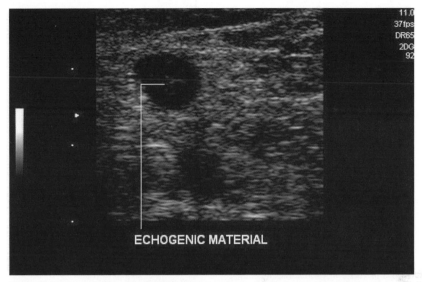

ECHOGENIC MATERIAL

Fig. 5.11 Deep vein thrombosis (DVT): note intraluminal echogenic material.

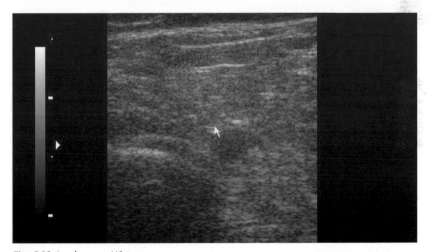

Fig. 5.12 Inadequate US image.

Positives and negatives

- Normal saphenofemoral confluence: no compression (Fig. 5.4) and compression (Fig. 5.5)
- Normal distal thigh: no compression (Fig. 5.6) and compression (Fig. 5.7)
- Normal popliteal: no compression (Fig. 5.8) and compression (Fig. 5.9)
- DVT (Figs 5.10 and 5.11)
- Inadequate image (Fig. 5.12).

49

Handy hints

✔ Strictly speaking, three-point compression US requires that only the groin, mid-thigh and popliteal fossa be scanned, because veins distal to a DVT usually are non-compressible. However, a common sense approach is to scan as much of the femoral vein as possible.

✔ Use plenty of gel.

✔ Press lightly to avoid obliterating the venous lumen (particularly in the popliteal fossa).

✔ A Valsalva manoeuvre may help to identify the femoral vein if there is any doubt. The normal response is a 15% increase in venous diameter on straining. (This also excludes occlusive thrombus in the iliac veins; however, the response will be less marked in a patient with congestive heart failure (CCF).)

✔ When progressing down the thigh, depth and focus may need to be increased.

✔ In obese patients, it may be necessary to use the lower-frequency (abdominal) probe, as the high-frequency probe loses resolution at depth.

✔ If the popliteal vein cannot be seen easily in the decubitus position, then scan the vein again with the patient seated or standing up.

✔ Patients with previous venous disease including DVT may have incompressible veins, resulting in a false-positive result.

✔ Up to 35% of the population have duplex popliteal veins. Ensure that this segment particularly is well visualized, to avoid false-negative results.

✔ If any segment cannot be adequately visualized, then call the study inadequate and refer to the radiology department.

What three-point compression ultrasound can tell you

• The presence or absence of proximal DVT, i.e. popliteal vein and above.

What three-point compression ultrasound can't tell you

• Presence or absence of *calf* vein DVT
• The likelihood of propagation or thromboembolism
• The cause of the pain if US is normal.

Now what?

• Proximal DVT: treat as per local treatment protocols.
• No proximal DVT:
  • patients with a high risk of *below-knee* DVT and normal proximal veins should probably be re-scanned at 48 hours to 1 week to rule out propagation of DVT.
  • other patients should be reassessed for other causes of their presentation.
• Inadequate scan: refer to Radiology and consider treatment for DVT in the interim period.

Summary

→ Three-point compression US is a useful investigation, which can diagnose proximal DVT quickly and accurately.

→ This timely diagnosis can improve patient flow in both the Emergency and Radiology Departments.

Chapter 6

The painful hip

Richard Wright, Sean McGovern

The question: is there a hip effusion?

Atraumatic hip pain is a common presenting symptom in children and can be caused by a number of inflammatory and infectious diseases. The detection of fluid within the hip joint is difficult clinically and notoriously unreliable with plain film radiography but relatively straightforward with focused ultrasound (US).

Atraumatic hip pain is much less common in adults. US can be used to detect fluid in children, with the proviso that different depth settings and probe (e.g. 4–7 MHz) may be necessary.

Why use US?

- *Diagnosis.* US uses no ionizing radiation, is cheap and takes only minutes to perform. Accurate reproducible measurements of effusion size are possible. Older children think that this is a cool test—no needles!
- *Localization and drainage.* US can be used to guide aspiration of the collection.
- *Other joints.* Although clinical identification and aspiration via the landmark technique is sufficient for large effusions in other joints, e.g. knee, US localization is useful for small effusions and in the obese.

Clinical picture

The child with a painful hip usually presents with a limp. There may be associated pyrexia. It is sometimes difficult to be sure which side is affected and rarely the presentation will be bilateral. A variety of conditions cause atraumatic hip pain in paediatric patients including:

- septic arthritis
- transient synovitis
- Perthes' disease
- slipped capital femoral epiphysis (SCFE).

Before you scan

- Explain to the child and parents the need for the procedure and obtain informed consent.
- Place the patient supine on a couch.
- Distraction techniques for the young child may be helpful. Subdued background lighting is desirable. Ask the parents or guardians to assist. Let the child hold the probe for a few moments at the start to reassure them. (Don't let them drop it!)
- Exposure of the hip area is necessary but the undergarment/diaper should usually be retained.

The technique and views

Patient's position

- Ideal: supine with hips in the neutral position without flexion (Fig. 6.1).
- However, it is more important to keep the child still than to obtain positioning perfection. If the child is reluctant to straighten the hip fully, ensure that both hips are examined in exactly the same position.
- This is a completely different technique from that used to identify DDH (developmental dysplasia of hip). This can cause confusion.

 Both hips must be examined in the same position with the legs as straight as is comfortable.

Probe and scanner settings

1. High-frequency (7–12 MHz) linear array probe.
2. Many scanners will have pre-set factors for paediatric hip. If not, use up to three focal spots set with the deepest spot just on the bone surface, usually a few centimetres deep.
3. Adjust the gain so that the soft tissues are relatively dark to allow visualization of a 'black' effusion.

Probe placement and landmarks

1. Scan the hip in a ventral, oblique plane along the long axis of the femoral neck (Fig. 6.1).
2. You should be able to identify (Fig. 6.2):
   - the brightly echogenic cortex of the femoral head and neck
   - the anterior margin of the acetabulum
   - the echolucent physis (growth plate)

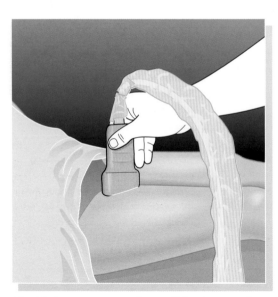

Fig. 6.1 *Patient supine, probe parallel to long axis femoral neck.*

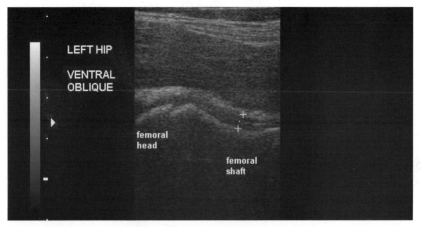

Fig. 6.2 *Normal hip joint, ventral oblique view, landmarks labelled, measurement calipers in situ.*

- the iliopsoas muscle superficial to the joint capsule
- the anterior recess of the normal joint capsule, its anterior and posterior margins parallel ('tram tracking')
- the normal capsule has a *concave contour* and its thickness (measured from the outer margin to the cortex of the femoral neck) measures 2–5 mm.
3. Measure at the widest point at 90° to the bony cortex using electronic calipers (Fig. 6.2).
4. Compare the two sides. The hip capsules' depth should be symmetric to within 2 mm of each other.
5. Pathology. When there is an effusion, one or more of the following will be observed (Fig. 6.3):
   - anechoic fluid distends capsule: convex margin, loss of 'tram tracking'
   - capsule depth greater than 5 mm;

- asymmetry: the affected joint's capsular depth will be more than 2 mm deeper than the normal side.

Note. In infants, clearly the upper limit of normal capsule depth will be less than 5 mm. In such cases, convexity and asymmetry are used as indicators of effusion.

Septic joints may contain echogenic debris but some septic joints will be clear and many joints with debris are not infected. This is *not* a reliable sign.

Arthrocentesis

Not all effusions require aspiration. Decision to aspirate depends on the clinical picture and other investigations (see below: *Now what?*). Joint aspiration can be performed in the ED, operating theatre (OT) or in the Radiology Department depending on the patient and local practice.

If aspirating the joint, you will require:

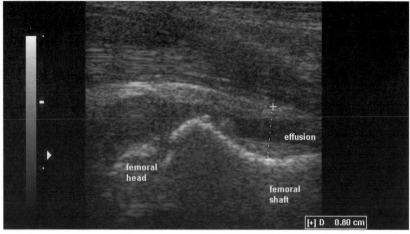

Fig. 6.3 *Hip effusion.*

- explanation and informed consent;
- a co-operative patient—this may entail local anaesthetic and/or conscious sedation (with appropriate medical assistance and monitoring) or even general anaesthetic in the OT
- sterile technique, sterile US probe sheath and gel (see also Chs 7 and 9)
- suitable needle and syringe
- specimen jars for laboratory analysis of the fluid.

The technique of US-guided hip-joint aspiration is similar to that used for draining effusions (Ch. 9). Introduce the needle along the long axis of the probe and perpendicular to the skin. Identify the needle (or its 'ring-down' artefact) on the US image, monitor the needle's progress into the collection and aspirate.

Essential views

One view of each hip identically positioned (in practice take three of each and use the best one).

Positives and negatives

- Normal hip joint (Fig. 6.2)
- Effusion (Fig. 6.3)
- Inadequate image (Fig. 6.4).

Handy hints

✔ Compare both sides (Fig. 6.5). Scan the asymptomatic side first to gain the child's trust.

✔ Beware bilateral joint effusion.

✔ Measure depth *perpendicular* to the cortex. Measurement at an angle will overestimate depth (Fig. 6.6).

 Both hips must be examined in the same position with the legs as straight as is comfortable.

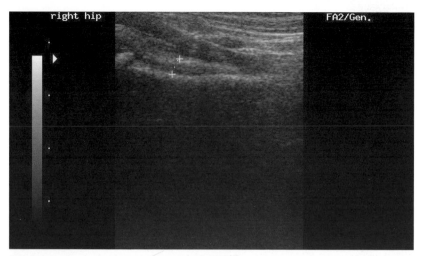

Fig. 6.4 *Inadequate view.*

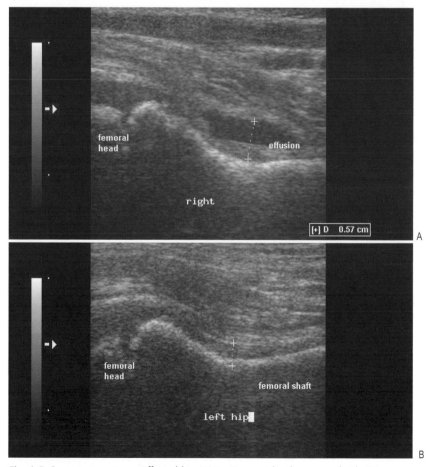

Fig. 6.5 *Comparative views. Affected hip (A) is >2 mm wider than normal side (B).*

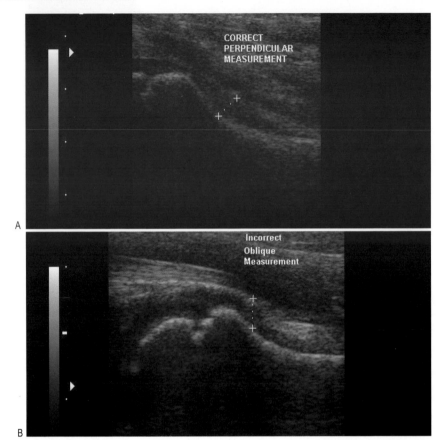

Fig. 6.6 *(A) Correct depth measurement (perpendicular to cortex) and (B) incorrect (angled) measurement.*

What US can tell you

- Is there an effusion? US accuracy is >90%.

What US can't tell you

- The cause of the effusion. Occasionally the 'slip' of a slipped capital femoral epiphysis (SCFE) may be seen or fragmentation of the femoral head in Perthes' disease. These, however, are late signs and their absence is not helpful. If fluid analysis is required, needle aspiration must be carried out.

However, US is useful when analysed together with clinical findings and other investigations such as white cell count.

- Is there an infection? A negative scan makes septic arthritis very unlikely but does not exclude *osteomyelitis*.

Now what?

- No effusion on US: look for other cause of presentation.
- Inadequate scan: repeat and reassess patient.

- Effusion on US: further investigations (e.g. blood tests, plain X-ray, magnetic resonance imaging) and management depend on clinical features and local practice.
- Aspiration of the effusion is often unnecessary: for example, in a child with a clinical and laboratory picture of improving transient synovitis.
- Joint aspiration can be performed in the ED, operating theatre or in the Radiology Department depending on the patient and local practice.

 Not all hip effusions require aspiration.

Summary

→ US can quickly, safely and reliably identify hip effusions.

→ A single adequate view of each hip is all that is required.

→ The identification or exclusion of an effusion helps guide patient management.

→ US can be used to guide joint aspiration.

Chapter 7

Central venous access

Justin Bowra

Why use ultrasound?

- In an emergency, it is vital to obtain vascular access rapidly and safely.
- Blind insertion of a central vein cannula (CVC), also known as the landmark technique, can be dangerous and technically difficult for many reasons such as cardiac arrest, intravascular depletion and abnormal anatomy.
- US-guided insertion of a CVC is best practice. It enables accurate location of the central vein, identifies anatomical variants and venous thrombosis and decreases the risk of complications such as damage to nearby structures. Several studies have demonstrated that insertion of a CVC using two-dimensional (2D) US guidance is safer and more successful than the landmark technique.
- In the UK, current National Institute for Clinical Excellence (NICE) guidelines (www.nice.org.uk) recommend 2D US guidance for emergency and elective CVC cannulation.
- US guidance may also be used when cannulating peripheral veins (such as the long saphenous vein) and arteries.

Anatomy

- The *internal jugular vein* (IJV) runs in the carotid sheath, usually lateral to the common carotid artery (CCA) and deep to the sternocleidomastoid muscle (SCM) (Fig. 7.1). Its compressibility and relative safety make it a preferred CVC site in the Emergency Department (ED). A traditional cannulation site is approximately halfway between the sternal notch and the mastoid process, at the bifurcation of the SCM.
- As well as compressibility, the *femoral vein* (FV, also known as *common femoral vein*) has the advantage of distance from important structures such as the airway and lungs. In the femoral sheath it is usually medial to the pulsation of the femoral artery, which lies approximately halfway between the symphysis pubis and the anterior superior iliac spine (ASIS) (Fig. 7.2; see also Ch. 5: *Deep vein thrombosis*).
- Subclavian vein cannulation is technically difficult and beyond the scope of this text.

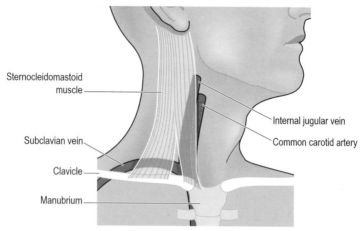

Fig. 7.1 *Relations of the right IJV, patient's head turned to left. IJV and CCA are deep to the sternocleidomastoid muscle.*

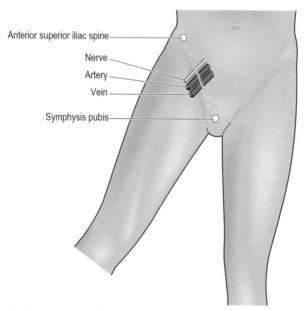

Fig. 7.2 *Relations of the right femoral vein. Patient's leg abducted.*

- It is essential to distinguish between veins and arteries on US:
  1. Vein larger, oval cross section, thinner walled and compressible (unless thrombus or proximal obstruction, for example massive pulmonary embolism (PE));
  2. Vein's diameter changes with respiration and Valsalva;
  3. Arterial pulsation (beware transmitted venous pulsation);
  4. Doppler waveform analysis will further differentiate vein from artery. However, Doppler is not essential and not recommended by NICE.

Which technique?

Three techniques are described. A combination of all three is used by the author.

'Static' technique

US is used to identify the target vein and mark the optimum site of needle entry prior to sterile preparation of the field. This confirms venous depth, course and compressibility. It is recommended as a 'screening exam' prior to using one of the other techniques below. Used alone, it is less technically demanding and obviates any requirement for sterility. However, it is not as safe as real-time US guidance.

Real-time transverse section (TS) and longitudinal section (LS)

Described below, both techniques require sterile probe and gel. Both are more difficult than the static technique and an assistant is recommended when first using either technique. However, real-time US guidance is safer than the static approach.

 US may be used to mark the site for subsequent cannulation, following which the probe is removed. However, real-time US guidance is safer.

CVC cannulation using real-time US: preparation

- Informed consent unless emergency.
- Patient attached to monitors. Local anaesthetic and Seldinger technique equipment.
- Choose site and confirm anatomy with static US, then prep and drape site.
- Prepare the probe with standard gel, then insert the probe into a sterile US probe sheath and apply sterile gel over the sheath (Fig. 7.3). A sterile glove may be used instead. An assistant will be required for this step.
- Although not essential, an assistant to hold the probe is helpful when you are inexperienced with this technique.
- US monitor in your line of sight: it is difficult and potentially hazardous to insert a CVC when craning to look over your shoulder at the screen.

Patient's position

- Dictated by clinical picture.
- IJV cannulation: 10° Trendelenburg tilt will significantly increase IJV diameter and prevent intracranial air embolism.
- Femoral cannulation: leg abducted.

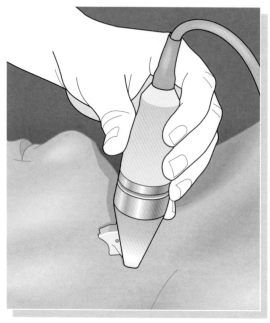

Fig. 7.3 *Initial probe placement IJV to confirm suitability for cannulation.*

Probe and scanner settings

- High-frequency (e.g. 7.5 MHz) linear array probe. Some probes have a notch in their midline to guide the needle.
- Focus depth 3 cm, depth setting 5 cm.

Technique

Transverse section (TS)

1. With your non-dominant hand, place probe transversely over the chosen site. Identify vein, artery and nearby structures on screen (Figs 7.4–7.7). Lymph nodes may mimic vessels in cross section but are not compressible or tubular.

2. Move probe and alter image depth and focus so that vein appears in the centre of the screen (Figs 7.7 and 7.8). This will serve as a landmark for vein position.

3. Administer local anaesthetic (LA) over the course of the vein at the probe's midway point (Fig. 7.9). When LA has taken effect, a scalpel may be used to nick the skin to ease the subsequent passage of the introducer needle. This step is not essential.

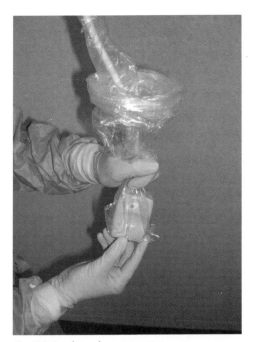

Fig. 7.4 *Sterile probe preparation.*

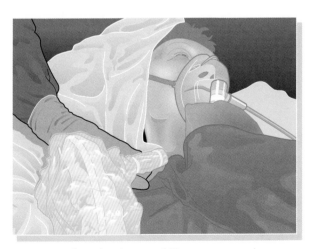

Fig. 7.5 *Sterile probe placement IJV, patient prepped.*

63

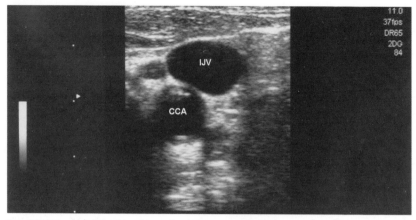

Fig. 7.6 *US image TS: IJV, CCA and nearby structures. IJV is compressed by probe pressure.*

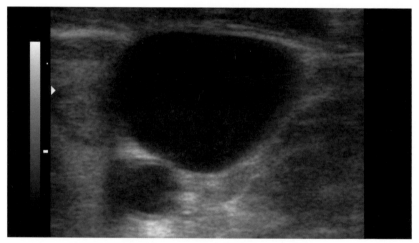

Fig. 7.7 *US image TS: IJV diameter enlarges with Valsalva manoeuvre.*

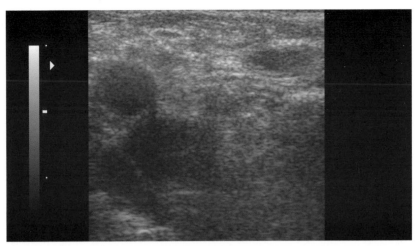

Fig. 7.8 US image TS: poorly focused, gain set too high and not centred on vein.

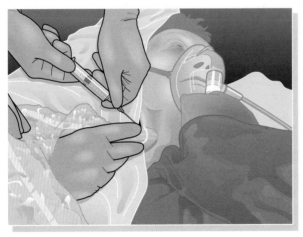

Fig. 7.9 Needle insertion using real time US guidance. Assistant holds probe.

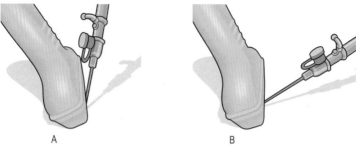

A   B

Fig. 7.10 *A. Correct: steep needle insertion with projected needle path intersecting vein in the plane of US image. B. Incorrect: needle directly touching probe. Needle tip will overshoot US plane.*

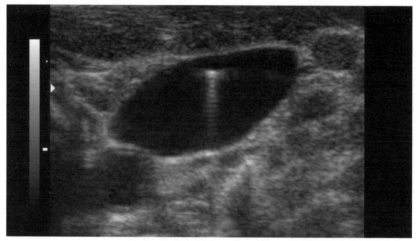

Fig. 7.11 *US image TS: 'ring-down' artefact demonstrates needle in vein.*

4. With your dominant hand, insert introducer needle (attached to syringe) at the site of LA, at a *steeper angle* to the skin than that used for blind CVC insertion. Introduce the needle at an angle and position to ensure that the needle tip intersects the vein *in the plane of the US image* and does not overshoot the plane of the US image (Fig. 7.10). Using TS method, the image of the needle often is not seen, but its 'ring-down' artefact will confirm its

position (Fig. 7.11). If in doubt, change the angle of the probe until the needle is seen (Fig. 7.12).

5. The major risk of such a steep angle is inadvertent 'through and through' venous puncture. Avoid this by the following:

- Introduce the needle more slowly than when performing blind CVC insertion.
- Introduce the needle under real-time visualization of the US image.

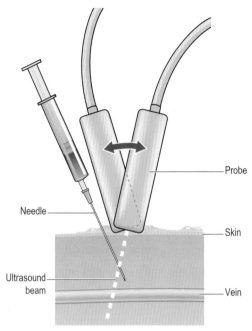

Probe

Needle

Skin

Ultrasound
beam

Vein

Fig. 7.12 *Changing the probe's angle until needle is visualized.*

- Watch for 'tenting' of the vein's upper wall inwards as the needle approaches the vein (Fig. 7.13). When the needle enters the vein, this tenting will diminish even if you do not see the needle in the vein. The needle tip (or its artefact) should be visible in the venous lumen (Fig. 7.14) but may not be if the US plane does not intersect the needle.
- Confirm position by aspirating venous blood.
- Once the needle has entered the vein, decrease the angle of the needle. Take care to ensure that the needle tip remains in the lumen.

6. Remove the syringe and introduce the guide wire. The guide wire should be visible in the venous lumen (Figs 7.15 and 7.16). Using transverse and longitudinal scanning, trace the path of the guide wire to ensure that it has not kinked back.
7. Remove the probe, complete Seldinger insertion of the CVC and check position with X-ray as per local protocol.

Longitudinal section (LS) method
1. Step 1 as for TS.
2. Once vein is identified, *rotate* the probe until the vein appears in LS: confirm that the vessel is venous using the checklist above ('Anatomy') (Fig. 7.17).

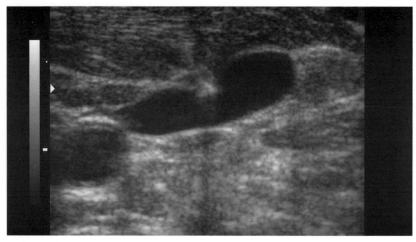

Fig. 7.13 US image TS: upper wall of vein 'tenting' as needle approaches.

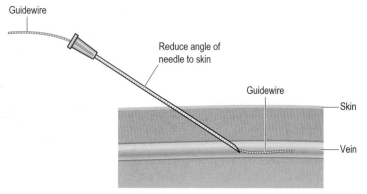

Fig. 7.14 Needle angle decreased, guide wire in vein.

3. Administer LA beneath the probe and consider nicking the skin with a scalpel as above.

4. Introduce introducer needle at a *shallow angle* as for traditional blind cannulation. This allows easier visualization of the needle on US (Fig. 7.18).

5. The major pitfall of this technique is inadvertently moving the probe so that its plane no longer *parallels* that of the vein and needle. This may lead to needle overshoot or even arterial cannulation.

6. Once the needle has entered the vein, complete steps 6 and 7 as above.

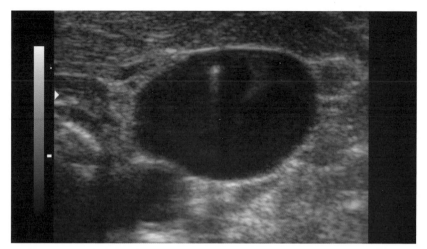

Fig. 7.15 US image TS: guide wire in vein.

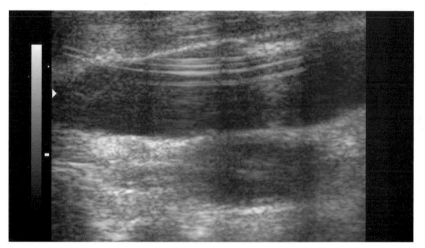

Fig. 7.16 US image LS: central line visible in lumen. Note ring-down.

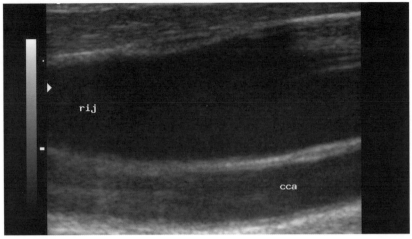

Fig. 7.17 US image LS: rij and cca. Vein is more superficial, wider lumen, thinner walls.

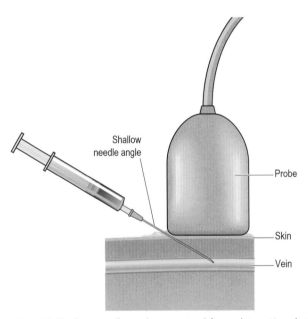

Fig. 7.18 Shallow needle angle is required for real time LS technique.

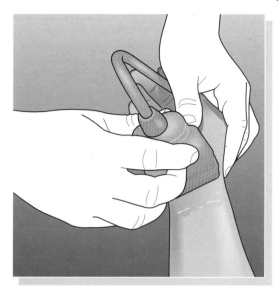

Fig. 7.19 Identifying radial artery on US.

TS technique vs. LS technique

TS technique
→ *Steep* angle needle entry.
→ Easier and preferred by most operators.
→ Difficult to visualize US image of needle: 'ring down' artefact used instead.
→ Risk of overshoot if probe plane does not *intersect* needle.

LS technique
→ *Shallow* angle needle entry
→ Easier to visualize needle
→ Risks if probe's plane no longer *parallels* that of the vein or needle: needle overshoot, arterial cannulation.

A combination of all three techniques (e.g. non-sterile screening exam, then TS to introduce needle and LS to confirm guide wire) is probably safest.

Handy hints and pitfalls

✔ Doppler is not required to distinguish veins from arteries.
✔ Keep the US screen directly in front, in your line of sight.
✔ When first using this technique, an assistant can be helpful.
✔ Needle angle differs between TS and LS techniques.
✔ Avoid through-and-through venous puncture by:
  ✔ slow needle insertion
  ✔ real-time US visualization
  ✔ watch for tenting of vein as needle approaches
  ✔ continuous aspiration of syringe
  ✔ decreasing the needle angle once it has entered the vein.
✔ US guidance may also be used when cannulating peripheral veins (such as the long saphenous vein) and arteries (Fig. 7.19).

Summary

→ US-guided CVC insertion is best practice and decreases the risk of complications.

→ The technique can be difficult to learn at first.

 Real-time US guidance is safer than simply using US to mark the site for subsequent cannulation.

 In addition, all the usual risks, contraindications and complications of Seldinger CVC insertion apply.

Chapter 8

Soft-tissue foreign bodies

Michael Hyland, Russell McLaughlin

The question: is there a foreign body?

To answer this question one must first employ the basic principles of history and examination followed by investigation. The question may be answered at any stage in this process. However, a foreign body (FB) can be missed at any stage in this process and no single Emergency Department (ED) investigation is universally applicable. Do not stray from the binary question: 'FB: yes or no?' Use of ultrasound (US) to diagnose other causes of soft-tissue symptoms is best left to a practitioner with extended training.

Why use US?

US is extremely useful for identifying or excluding soft-tissue FB not readily visible on X-ray, such as wood, plastic or aluminium. Once identified, US can aid in the removal of an FB.

Clinical picture

The patient can usually remember the injury and describe the suspected FB and how it entered the skin. History may not be complete in certain situations (for example in paediatric and delayed presentations). Despite negative investigations, a patient complaining of persisting FB sensation or ongoing wound infection should be assumed to have an FB until proven otherwise.

The technique and views

Patient's position

- Dictated by clinical picture
- FB in hand/forearm: seated, resting both forearms on examination couch
- FB torso/lower limb: supine or prone.

Probe and scanner settings

- Superficial FB: high-frequency probe (10–15 MHz) with a thick layer of sterile transducer gel
- Stand-off pad or sterile glove filled with water will improve the image by bringing the *superficial* tissues into the probe focal zone (Figs 8.1 and 8.2)
- Deeper FB: 5–7.5 MHz linear array transducer is most useful

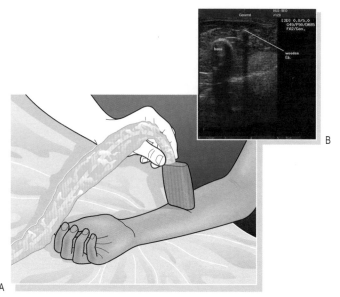

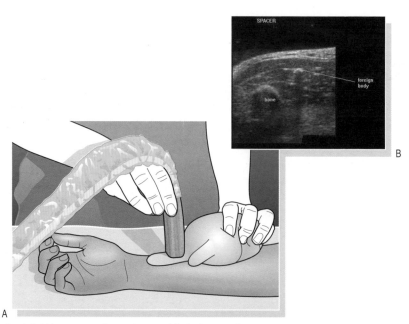

Fig. 8.1 (A) Linear probe on patient's forearm. (B) US image: loss of near field.

Fig. 8.2 (A) Linear probe and water filled glove on forearm. (B) US image: near field.

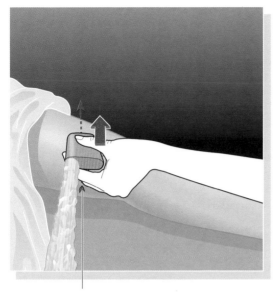

Entry point of foreign body

Fig. 8.3 *Scanning along FB track.*

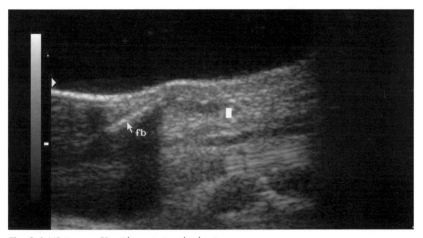

Fig. 8.4 *US image: FB with posterior shadowing.*

- Focus and depth setting depends on suspected FB depth.

Probe placement and landmarks
- Scan along the suspected FB track (Fig. 8.3).

- FBs are usually hyper-echoic and often demonstrate posterior shadowing if they are sufficiently dense (Fig. 8.4). They may be surrounded by hypo-echoic fluid due to haematoma or abscess.

75

- If an abnormality or FB is identified repeat the scan with the probe rotated through 90° and confirm that it conforms to the shape of the suspected FB. Also note if there is more than one FB or if a single piece of wood has broken into several fragments.
- If in doubt about the nature of an identified structure, then scan the same area on the other limb to exclude a normal anatomical structure.
- When an FB is identified, mark it at the skin surface and note any adjacent anatomy, such as vessels, joints or tendons, which may be important during subsequent surgical removal.
- Occasionally needle localization is required to aid removal of an FB. Obtain informed consent, clean the skin with antiseptic and use sterile technique, sterile gel and probe sheath.
  1. Prepare with local anaesthetic.
  2. Scan along the suspected FB track. Introduce a fine needle (e.g. 25G) through the skin so that the needle tip or its artefact is visible on the image. Slowly advance the needle until it is in contact with the FB. The needle can then be used to direct surgical intervention.
  3. It may be tempting to attempt real-time removal of a foreign body under US guidance; however, the authors find this impractical for the following reasons:
- incising along the wound track introduces air into the soft tissues, obscuring the US image;
- scanning and performing the removal simultaneously can be awkward and requires four hands rather than two.

Handy hints

✔ Use a stand-off pad or sterile glove filled with water to improve view of *superficial* tissues.

✔ If in doubt about the nature of an identified structure, then scan the same area on the other limb to exclude a normal anatomical structure.

✔ Mark the position of the FB with a pen or needle to aid in subsequent removal.

What US can tell you

- Whether an FB is present;
- Position of FB;
- Presence of multiple FBs;
- Presence of nearby structures, for example tendons, vessels.

What US can't tell you

- What the FB is;
- Nature of the surrounding fluid.

 Believe the patient and not the scan. If the patient says that an FB is present it usually is.

Now what?

History or examination suggests FB

- *US positive.* Consider FB removal after evaluating symptoms and proximity of important anatomical structures.
- *US negative.* Consider repeating US and evaluating symptoms in approximately 1–2 weeks. Alternatively, discuss with radiologist regarding further imaging.
- *US positive but undetectable at operation.* Repeat US and guide needle to FB in wound. Dissect along needle toward FB.

Do not attempt to remove an FB just because it is there. Always consider the patient's wishes and symptoms and the local anatomy.

Summary

→ US is useful for identifying a soft-tissue FB.

→ US can identify an FB not seen on plain radiographs.

→ US can aid the removal of an FB.

→ US is not an alternative to history and physical examination.

Chapter 9

Draining pleural effusions and ascites

Michael Hyland, Justin Bowra

Why use ultrasound?

Diagnosis

- US will identify small pleural effusions missed by CXR (chest X-ray).
- US diagnosis of ascites is rapid, safe, more reliable than clinical diagnosis and does not expose the patient to radiation.

Localization and drainage

- US can then be used to guide aspiration of the collection safely.

Handy hints and pitfalls

- ✔ Like all fluid collections, effusions are dark and hypo-echoic on US (Fig. 9.1) and demonstrate posterior acoustic enhancement.
- ✔ Bowel air and normal lung tissue reflect sound poorly and produce scatter (Fig. 9.2). Therefore, if you are unable to see clearly a dark fluid stripe, assume there is no effusion.
- ✔ Small particles within the collection suggest the presence of debris.
- ✔ Linear structures may be seen to subdivide the collection if it is multi-loculated.

- ✔ Failure to consider diaphragmatic movement with respiration may make thoracocentesis hazardous.
- ✔ Similarly, organomegaly and coagulopathy may make paracentesis hazardous.
- ✔ Coagulopathy may make either procedure hazardous.
- ✔ Real-time US guidance of aspiration is safer than merely using US to identify the optimum drainage site for later blind aspiration.

 If you cannot identify a dark fluid stripe, assume that there is no effusion.

 Thoracocentesis: consider diaphragmatic movement due to respiration.

 Paracentesis: consider organomegaly and coagulopathy.

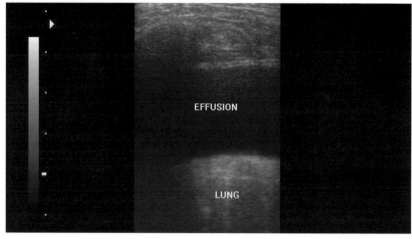

Fig. 9.1 *Intercostal view, pleural effusion with posterior acoustic enhancement. Linear array probe.*

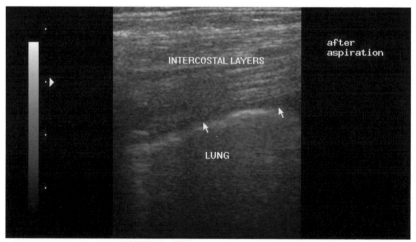

Fig. 9.2 *Intercostal view, effusion has been aspirated. A very small amount of fluid remains (arrows).*

Pleural effusions

Clinical picture

- Usual symptoms/signs: an effusion may not be symptomatic. However, clinically significant effusions should demonstrate dullness to percussion and diminished breath sounds on auscultation.

- Pitfalls: conditions which mimic pleural effusion clinically and on CXR include lobar collapse and elevated hemidiaphragm. US can distinguish these from pleural effusion.

Preparation
- Move the patient to the resuscitation area if required.
- Attach monitors and oxygen.

Sterile equipment
- Drapes, gloves, gown, dressing pack, antiseptic
- Probe sheath and lubricant
- Local anaesthetic (e.g. 1% lidocaine), needle, 5 ml syringe
- Large cannula-over-needle and scalpel blade (see step 8 below). Alternatives include large needle or dedicated aspiration kit and depend on local practice
- 3-way tap, large syringe, specimen containers.

Patient's position
- Easiest position: patient seated with arms folded, leaning forward (Fig. 9.3)
- If patient is unwell: semi-supine position.

Imaging the effusion
Probe and scanner settings
1. Standard curved probe may be used initially to confirm the presence of fluid and nearby anatomical structures. A smaller, 5–7.5 MHz array probe should then be used for a more accurate assessment of depth of the effusion.
2. Focus depth 3–7 cm.
3. Depth setting 10 cm.

Probe placement and landmarks
1. If patient seated, posterior approach: scan from the paravertebral muscles to the posterior axillary line (Fig. 9.3). If supine, begin in the mid-axillary line and sweep probe posteriorly.
2. Keep the probe parallel to the ribs and scan between them, through the intercostal muscles (Fig. 9.4).

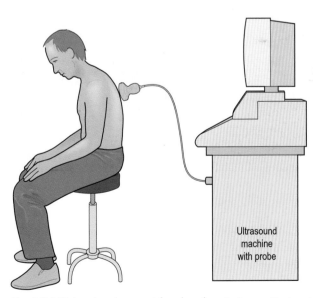

Ultrasound
machine
with probe

Fig. 9.3 *Initial probe placement for pleural aspiration: patient seated with arms folded, leaning forward. Resting the elbows on a pillow or a trolley will help the patient to maintain this position.*

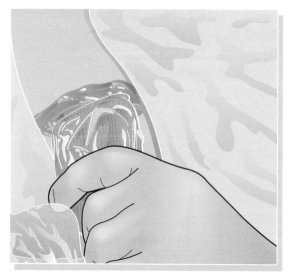

Fig. 9.4 Sterile probe and field, probe alignment parallel to ribs.

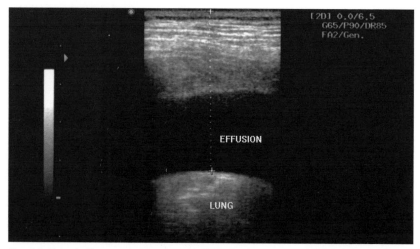

Fig. 9.5 Pleural effusion as in Fig. 9.1, depth measured.

3. Fluid will be readily visible in the pleural space. It is demarcated by the chest wall and visceral pleura (Fig. 9.1). Alter probe settings as required. Identify the extent of the effusion, position of relevant structures (e.g. liver) and diaphragmatic movement.

Essential views

At least one good view of the effusion must be obtained and recorded.

Positives and negatives

- Pleural effusion (Figs 9.1 and 9.5)
- Intercostal scan post-aspiration: a small amount of fluid remains (Fig. 9.2).

Draining the effusion: thoracocentesis

1. Identify a site two rib spaces below the top of the effusion, but well above the diaphragm. The site should be above a rib to avoid the neurovascular bundle and should be where the effusion is deepest.
2. Take into account diaphragmatic movement with respiration, to minimize risk of diaphragmatic/organ injury.
3. Measure the depth of the fluid (Fig. 9.5). This is particularly important, to prevent introducing the aspiration needle/cannula too deeply.
4. Mark the skin (pressure from the plastic cover of a needle is useful).
5. Using full aseptic technique clean the skin with antiseptic.
6. Administer local anaesthetic.
7. While the anaesthetic is taking effect, place the probe inside a sterile sheath and image the collection.
8. Incise the skin with a scalpel. (This step is optional but eases passage of the cannula.)
9. Introduce a needle with plastic sheath as above, along the long axis of the probe, perpendicular to the skin and through the incision. Identify the needle (or its 'ring-down' artefact, see Ch. 7) on the ultrasound image. Monitor the needle's progress into the collection.
10. Remove the needle, leaving the plastic cannula in situ.
11. Attach a three-way tap to the cannula and aspirate the collection. Send any necessary samples for laboratory assessment.
12. When no further fluid can be aspirated re-image the collection to assess its size. If fluid is still present, alter the cannula's position to allow further aspiration.
13. When no further fluid can be drained remove the cannula in expiration or during Valsalva manoeuvre to ensure positive intrathoracic pressure. Apply a dressing to the skin incision.
14. Many authorities recommend a maximum 1–1.5 L aspiration at any one time to avoid possible complications of pulmonary re-expansion and fluid shifts.

 Remember diaphragmatic movement due to respiration.

Ascites

Clinical picture
- The patient may have signs of chronic liver disease and may be coagulopathic.
- The abdomen is distended and may be tense. Shifting dullness may be present.
- Pitfalls/caveats: the liver may be enlarged or shrunken. The spleen may also be massively enlarged.

 Consider organomegaly and coagulopathy.

Preparation, equipment, probe and scanner settings
As for pleural effusions above.

The patient is usually supine. As in traumatic haemoperitoneum, small collections are best seen in Morison's pouch therefore right decubitus position may help.

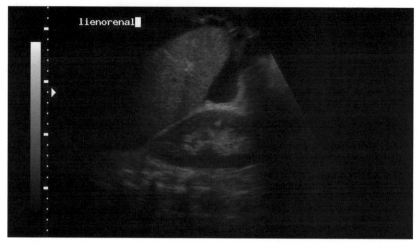

Fig. 9.6 *Ascites: large amount of free fluid below left hemidiaphragm and in the lienorenal angle.*

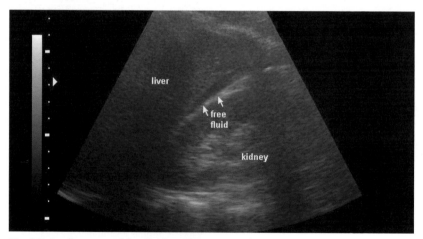

Fig. 9.7 *Small amount of free fluid in Morison's pouch.*

Imaging ascites

1. Scan the abdomen as for free fluid in trauma (Ch. 4, FAST).
2. Pay special attention to the following areas where fluid collects early in ascites:

- Morison's pouch and below both hemidiaphragms (Figs 9.6–9.8)
- The pelvis behind the bladder or uterus (see Fig. 4.15, page 36).

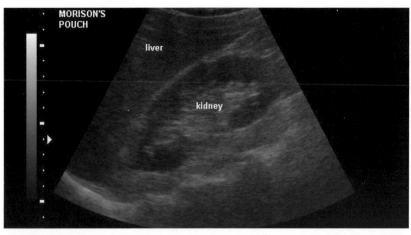

Fig. 9.8 Morison's pouch, no ascites.

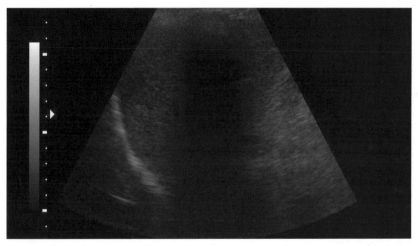

Fig. 9.9 Morison's pouch, inadequate view.

3. Save and print images confirming the presence of fluid with measurements of depth.

Essential views

At least one good view of the ascites must be obtained and recorded.

Positives and negatives

• Ascites (Figs 9.6 and 9.7)

• Negative scan: no ascites in Morison's pouch (Fig. 9.8)

• Inadequate image (Fig. 9.9).

Draining ascites: paracentesis

If drainage is being considered then the same procedure should be followed as for pleural effusion, with the following differences:

85

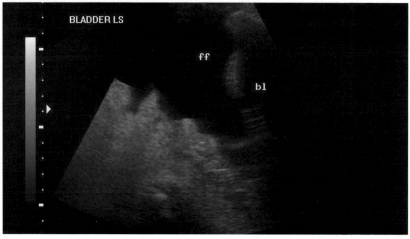

Fig. 9.10 *Suitable site for aspiration. ff = free fluid; bl = bladder.*

- Scan the collection thoroughly and measure the fluid collection's diameter in two planes. Ensure that you do not mistake fluid within structures such as gall bladder for free fluid.
- Identify a site with no bowel between the abdominal wall and the fluid and no nearby organs (Fig. 9.10).
- Traditionally, the left iliac fossa is recommended as the safest site for blind paracentesis, with a pillow under the right hip to allow fluid to collect on the left side. Real-time US guidance largely supplants this advice.

Draining effusions: summary

What US can tell you
- Is there a fluid collection?
- Is it accessible for drainage?
- Is it suitable for drainage? If there is much debris or the collection is multi-loculated it is probably unsuitable for complete drainage.

What US can't tell you
- The nature of the fluid: for example, haemothorax, empyema, transudate.

Complications of draining effusions
- Pain
- Pneumothorax
- Introduction of infection
- Perforation of nearby organs, for example diaphragm, lung, bowel
- Mistaking fluid within structures such as bladder for ascites
- Haemorrhage, due to vascular or organ injuries.

 If you cannot identify a dark fluid stripe with posterior acoustic enhancement, assume that there is no effusion.

Chapter 10

Shock and cardiac arrest

Justin Bowra, George Rudan

Why use ultrasound?

Diagnosis

Shock may be defined as a global state of inadequate tissue oxygenation. Its causes may be summarized as follows:

- cardiogenic (e.g. massive myocardial infarction)
- hypovolaemic (e.g. blood loss in trauma)
- distributive (e.g. sepsis, anaphylaxis)
- obstructive (e.g. massive pulmonary embolism (PE), pericardial tamponade)
- dissociative (e.g. cyanide poisoning).

Time is of the essence in commencing resuscitation and establishing a diagnosis in this setting. US may assist rapid identification of the following causes of shock:

- pericardial tamponade
- ruptured abdominal aortic aneurysm (AAA)
- massive pulmonary embolus (PE)
- hypovolaemia
- cardiogenic shock.

In the setting of **cardiac arrest**, US allows rapid differentiation of the following:

- pericardial tamponade
- hypovolaemia
- cardiac standstill.

Intervention

- US can be used to guide emergent pericardiocentesis in cardiac tamponade.
- US-guided CVC access: for CVP monitoring and delivery of fluids and inotropes.
- US-guided placement of intercostal catheter (e.g. in massive haemothorax) reduces the risk of incorrect placement.

Shock and cardiac arrest: scanning the patient

Preparation

- Move the patient to the resuscitation area.
- Attach monitors and oxygen and address ABCs.
- Get help: the doctor performing the scan should not also be resuscitating the patient.
- Arrested patient: arrest team and protocols as per local practice.
- If monitors demonstrate pulseless VT/VF, defibrillate as per guidelines.

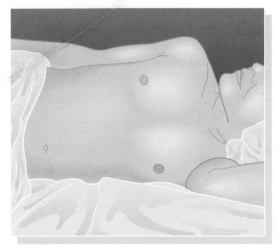

Fig. 10.1 *Patient in left lateral decubitus position.*

- If monitors demonstrate pulseless electrical activity (PEA) or asystole, proceed to US during breaks in cardiopulmonary resuscitation (CPR) for pulse checks. (Note: cardiac scan from the subxiphoid position often is possible during ongoing CPR.)
- Sterile equipment is ideal if performing US-guided intervention such as pericardiocentesis, but this must be balanced against the urgency of the situation. Many Emergency Departments (EDs) will have dedicated equipment for procedures such as pericardiocentesis.

 ED investigations (including US) must not delay resuscitation of a shocked or arrested patient.

Patient's position
- Dictated by clinical picture (e.g. arrested patient)
- Supine is most practical

- Cardiac scan: ideal position is left lateral, which brings the heart to the left of the sternum (hence less shadowing) and closer to the probe (Fig. 10.1). However, adequate scanning is still possible in supine or semi-recumbent position.

Probe and scanner settings
- It must be emphasized that the techniques described below are no substitute for formal echocardiography. Without formal training in echocardiography and dedicated equipment, echo-quality cardiac images are simply impossible and images generated with standard ED US machines must be interpreted with caution (Fig. 10.2).
- With this borne in mind, most ED US machines with standard curved low-frequency probes are capable of visualizing the heart and pericardium sufficiently to answer some of the basic questions listed below, particularly the presence of cardiac standstill and pericardial tamponade.

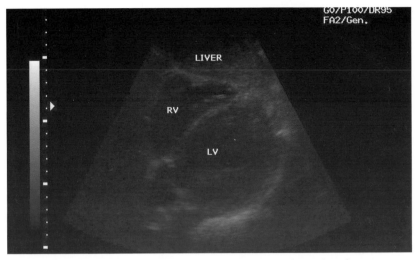

GO7P100/DR95
FA2/Gen.

LIVER

RV

LV

Fig. 10.2 *Normal heart. Standard ED US image, which lacks the quality of echocardiographic images.*

- Some ED US machines have Doppler and M-mode capability and a microconvex probe (small footprint minimizes rib artefact). All of these will assist in transthoracic scans of the heart and pericardium.
- For further tips, see *Handy hints and pitfalls* below.
- Transoesophageal echocardiography is beyond the scope of this text.
- For abdominal scans, use a standard low-frequency curved probe. Focus and depth should be dictated by patient's habitus and the region scanned.

Probe placement and landmarks

1. Cardiac scan: several probe positions are used. Three in particular are useful for the ED sonographer (see also Ch. 4, FAST):
   - left longitudinal parasternal (henceforth simply referred to as 'parasternal') (Fig. 10.3)
   - subxiphoid (also known as 'subcostal') (Fig. 10.4)
   - apical: probe placed at the apex beat and angled towards the right scapula (Fig. 10.5).

While any may suffice for identification of pericardial fluid or cardiac standstill, a combination is required to visualize the heart more fully (e.g. to comment on left ventricular motion). Sliding the probe down from the parasternal and across to the apical window will also assist in complete visualization.

Several other 'windows' are used by echocardiographers and include right parasternal and suprasternal. These are beyond the scope of this book.

Look for the following in particular:

- Pericardial fluid: this most commonly appears as a black stripe around the heart (Figs 4.4 and 10.6). However, its appearance is determined by its nature: for example, clotted blood will demonstrate a density similar to that of soft tissue.

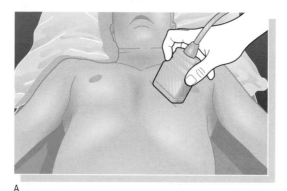

A

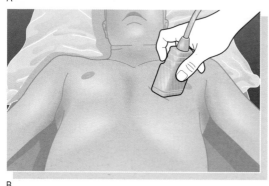

B

Fig. 10.3 *Probe in left longitudinal parasternal position. (A) Long axis orientation. (B) Short axis orientation.*

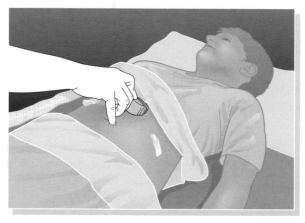

Fig. 10.4 *Probe in subxiphoid position. Shallow angle is required to visualize the heart and pericardium adequately.*

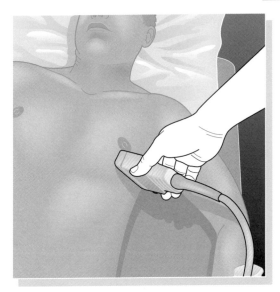

Fig. 10.5 Probe in apical position, angled towards right scapula.

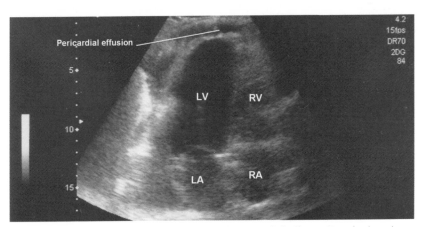

Fig. 10.6 Apical four-chamber view of heart with pericardial effusion. Standard quality achievable with emergency US. LV = left ventricle; RV = right ventricle; LA = left atrium; RA = right atrium.

- As noted in Chapter 4, in true cardiac tamponade the pressure of the tamponade on the right ventricle (RV) impairs RV filling during diastole and the RV collapses (Fig. 10.7). However, this can be difficult to assess for the non-echocardiographer, and false-positive findings of pericardial fluid may be seen in the presence of pleural fluid or an anterior fat pad.

91

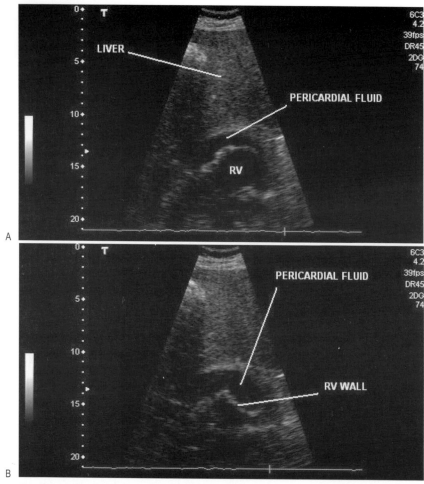

Fig. 10.7 Subxiphoid US images of tamponade, liver used as acoustic window. (A) Systole; RV = right ventricle. (B) Diastole, same patient: RV collapse.

- False negatives may occur in the presence of localized or loculated pericardial effusions, which may be missed by US.
- Hence, scan cautiously and through as many views as possible (see below) to rule out false positives and negatives.

- If US appears to demonstrate pericardial fluid, ascertain whether it surrounds the heart completely and, if time permits, arrange urgent bedside echocardiogram while preparing for pericardiocentesis.
- Cardiac standstill: in the arrested patient with PEA/asystole, this carries an extremely poor prognosis.

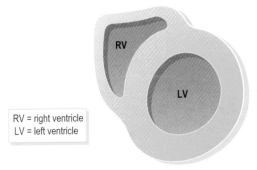

RV = right ventricle
LV = left ventricle

Fig. 10.8 *Cross-section of heart demonstrating relative thickness of LV and RV.*

- Hyperkinetic heart: in the absence of arrhythmia or acute valve disease (particularly acute mitral regurgitation), cardiogenic shock is unlikely if the heart is beating strongly. Assess the patient for hypovolaemia or causes of high-output states such as anaemia and thyrotoxicosis.
- Left ventricular (LV) hypokinesis: this can be difficult to assess for the non-cardiologist. The LV is seen behind the RV on a parasternal view and is much thicker-walled. The relative strength and wall thickness of the LV usually give it a convex shape on US and cause it to push forward into the thinner-walled RV (Fig. 10.8). The normal LV contracts symmetrically in systole. If one wall is seen **not** to move inwards during systole then myocardial infarction may be the cause of the patient's picture (cardiogenic shock).
- If the **entire** LV is dilated and contracting poorly, consider causes of global hypokinesis (cardiomyopathy) such as viral, idiopathic and alcoholic cardiomyopathy or severe sepsis.

- Right ventricle (RV): this lies in front of the LV, appears smaller on US and has an irregular shape. Like the LV, the RV should contract forcefully during systole and fill during diastole. Although RV changes may occur with conditions such as massive PE, even experienced echocardiographers find that the RV is difficult to assess. This is because of its irregular shape and acoustic shadowing from the overlying sternum. Examination of the inferior vena cava (IVC) is easier (see below).

 Avoid attempting more than a rough description of ventricular appearance and function. Over-interpretation of poor quality images is dangerous. Formal assessment is complex and requires calculations, equipment and experience not possessed by ED sonographers.

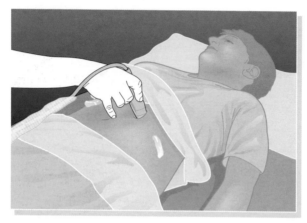

Fig. 10.9 *Initial probe position for assessment of abdominal aorta and inferior vena cava. Note different angle to that used for subxiphoid pericardial scan.*

2. Abdominal aorta and inferior vena cava (IVC): as for AAA scans (Ch. 3), place the probe in the subxiphoid position, angled directly posteriorly (Figs 3.3 and 10.9). Identify landmarks and differentiate between the aorta and IVC as described in Chapter 3. Look for the following in particular:

   • Abdominal aortic aneurysm (AAA): as previously noted, in a shocked patient assume that AAA is leaking or ruptured.

   • IVC distension and compressibility: normal IVC collapses with inspiration. Its cross-sectional area is greater than that of a normal aorta. If IVC is distended, not collapsing with inspiration and not easily compressed by direct pressure with the US probe, in a shocked patient this strongly suggests distal obstruction (Figs. 10.10 & 10.11). Potential causes include massive PE, tension pneumothorax and cardiac tamponade. However, bear in mind that there are many other causes for elevated caval pressure such as pulmonary hypertension.

   • Conversely, if IVC appears underfilled this strongly suggests hypovolaemia as the cause of the patient's shock.

3. Free fluid in thorax or abdomen: scan as for FAST (Ch. 4). Usually the clinical picture will have alerted the clinician to the presence of truncal trauma. However, atraumatic pleural effusions and ascitic collections may be associated with shock (e.g. empyema and spontaneous bacterial peritonitis). Large intrathoracic fluid collections may of themselves impair cardiorespiratory function, and massive ascites will impair diaphragmatic excursion (although the alert clinician should not require US to suspect the latter).

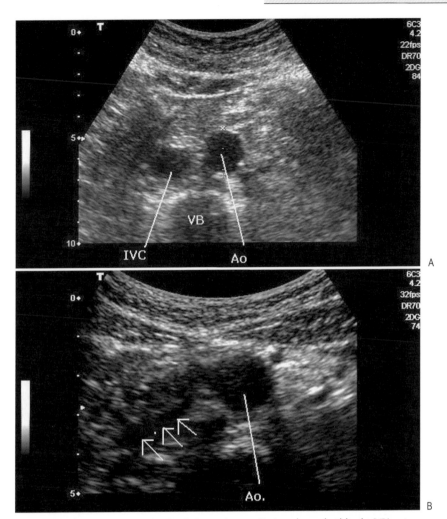

Fig. 10.10 Inferior vena cava (IVC), abdominal aorta (Ao) and vertebral body (VB), subxiphoid views. (A) Uncompressed. (B) Gentle pressure by probe: IVC compressed (arrows).

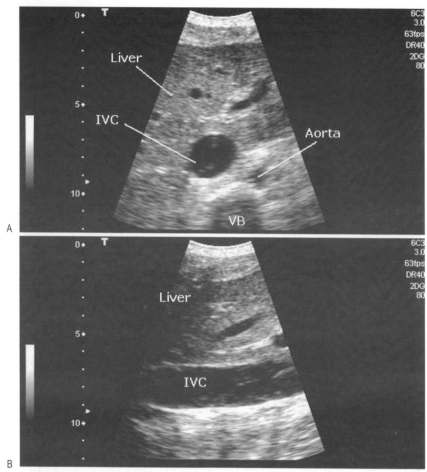

Fig. 10.11 Distended, non-compressible inferior vena cava (IVC) viewed using liver as acoustic window. (A) Transverse image. (B) Longitudinal image. Patient with pericardial tamponade. VB = vertebral body.

Positives and negatives

- Subxiphoid long axis view, normal heart (Fig. 10.12)
- Apical four chamber view, pericardial effusion (Fig. 10.6)
- Tamponade (Fig. 10.7)

- Inadequate cardiac image (Fig. 10.13)
- Compressible IVC (Fig. 10.10)
- Distended, non-compressible IVC (Fig. 10.11)
- Abdominal aorta and IVC, inadequate image (Fig. 10.14).

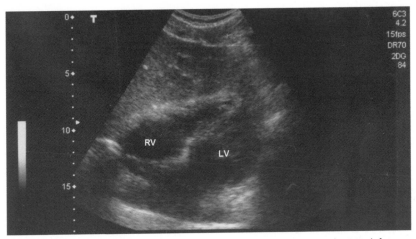

Fig. 10.12 Subxiphoid long axis view of normal heart. RV = right ventricle; LV = left ventricle.

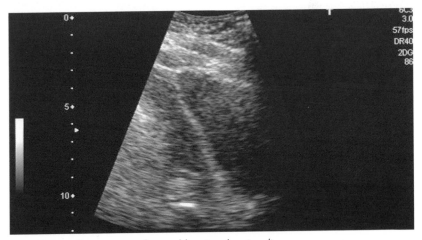

Fig. 10.13 Inadequate view of normal heart and pericardium.

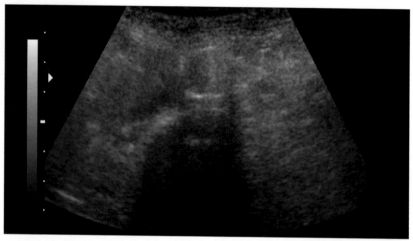

Fig. 10.14 *Inadequate image abdominal aorta and inferior vena cava. Round calcified structure probably represents abdominal aorta. Deeper structure with acoustic shadowing probably represents vertebral body.*

Handy hints and pitfalls

✔ Be aware of your own limitations: you are not a cardiologist! Avoid the temptation to comment on subtle or more complex pathology (such as valve disease) unless you have been trained formally in echocardiography (including M-mode).

✔ Similarly, the quality of cardiac images is much less than those generated by dedicated echocardiography machines. Over interpretation of poor quality images is dangerous.

✔ Tips to improve cardiac image quality:
  ✔ use the cardiac setting if your US machine has one
  ✔ decrease the gain (Ch. 2) and increase the contrast—this will sharpen the image
  ✔ if possible, altering the probe frequency may help to reduce artefact due to cardiac wall motion

  ✔ in a ventilated patient, temporarily turning off the positive end-expiratory pressure (PEEP) may improve images from all windows.

✔ ED sonographers trained in FAST are most comfortable with a subxiphoid view of the heart, and any of the three cardiac windows described above **may** suffice for identification of pericardial fluid or cardiac standstill.

✔ However, no single window will yield adequate views in every patient. For example, in the obese the subxiphoid window yields poor cardiac views, and the parasternal window may yield poor results in emphysematous patients. Hence, it is wise to practise the other views described above at every opportunity.

✔ A combination of views is required to visualize the heart adequately (e.g. to comment on left ventricular motion).

✔ In the subxiphoid position, using the liver as an acoustic window may improve image quality. Hence, consider sliding the probe to the right of the xiphisternum and angle it towards the left shoulder.

✔ The RV can be difficult to assess even for cardiologists. Assessment of the IVC is easier.

✔ If in doubt regarding your findings, continue treatment on clinical grounds and consider more definitive investigation, e.g. urgent bedside echocardiogram.

Echocardiography: talking the talk

At times you will have to describe your US findings to a cardiologist (e.g. when requesting a formal echocardiogram to confirm abnormal findings). It is useful to understand a little of their terminology.

Types of US used in echocardiograms

• B-mode: the type used in emergency US to produce a two-dimensional (2D) scan plane (see Ch. 2).

• M-mode: 'motion' mode uses sound transmitted along a single line and displays movement (e.g. the motion of valves or the ventricular walls) plotted against time as 'waves' on the screen. It is beyond the scope of this chapter.

• Doppler scanning demonstrates flow of fluid (such as blood) in colour format. It can be used to assist in the differentiation of vessels from other fluid-filled structures.

Cardiac axis

Using the views described above, echocardiographers view and describe the heart in planes (Fig. 10.15):

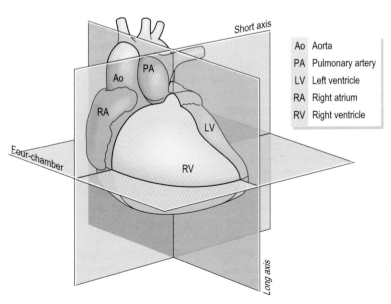

Ao	Aorta
PA	Pulmonary artery
LV	Left ventricle
RA	Right atrium
RV	Right ventricle

Fig. 10.15 The echocardiographic axes.

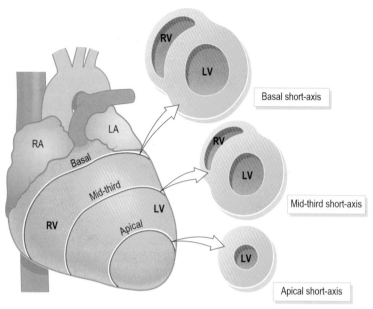

Fig. 10.16 *Series of short-axis views of heart.*

1. Long-axis view: this runs parallel to the heart's long axis. In the parasternal position (with probe marker pointing to patient's right shoulder) this allows simultaneous visualization of the LV and the outflow tract of the RV (Fig. 10.3A).
2. Short-axis view: perpendicular to the long axis (probe marker pointing to left shoulder in the parasternal position) (Fig. 10.3B). Sliding the probe (maintained in this position) along the long axis will allow a series of 'sectional' views of the LV and RV, which allows an assessment of relative wall thickness and contractility (Fig. 10.16).
3. Four-chamber view: the long-axis view which simultaneously demonstrates all four chambers. This is usually obtained from the apical window (Fig. 10.6) but may be obtained from the subxiphoid window.

It is important to note that these planes are **not** longitudinal or transverse with respect to the patient, as the heart itself is obliquely angled. While this may seem obvious, it represents a departure from the longitudinal and transverse windows described in this and other texts of emergency US.

Now what?

- Cardiac standstill in PEA or asystole: poor prognosis. Review decision to continue CPR.
- Pericardial fluid, clinical picture of tamponade: arrange urgent bedside echocardiography if possible. Prepare for pericardiocentesis.
- Small, hyperkinetic heart: suspect hypovolaemia. Continue fluid resuscitation and assess response.

- Gross LV hypokinesis: consider LV myocardial infarction or other causes of hypokinesis such as severe sepsis.
- IVC is distended and not easily compressed: suspect distal obstruction. Reassess patient for quickly reversible causes such as tension pneumothorax and cardiac tamponade. US may suggest PE but is inadequate for diagnosis, so if clinical picture suggests massive PE, decision to proceed to formal investigation (e.g. CT) or urgent thrombolysis depends on clinical picture.
- IVC underfilled: consider hypovolaemia. Continue fluid resuscitation and assess response.
- Unstable patient and AAA: notify surgical team immediately. The patient must be transferred immediately to OT for AAA repair.
- Massive pleural fluid collection causing cardiorespiratory compromise, whether traumatic (haemothorax) or atraumatic (e.g. malignancy-associated): urgent thoracocentesis via intercostal catheter.
- Unstable trauma patient and intra-abdominal free fluid (FF): immediate transfer to theatre for laparotomy.
- Inadequate scan: refer (e.g. for urgent echocardiogram) and continue resuscitation and treatment on clinical grounds.

 If in doubt about cardiac findings, refer to an echocardiographer.

Summary

→ Bedside US in the shocked or arrested patient is rapid, safe and allows ongoing resuscitation of the patient in the ED.

→ US assists rapid differentiation of many of the causes of shock but is not a substitute for formal echocardiography.

→ US can assist urgent interventions in the shocked/arrested patient such as pericardiocentesis and central venous access.

→ However, US and other ED investigations *must not delay* resuscitation.

→ If in doubt, continue treatment on clinical grounds and consider more definitive investigation, e.g. urgent bedside echocardiogram.

Chapter 11

Renal tract

Justin Bowra, Stella McGinn

Introduction

Ureteric colic, acute renal failure (ARF) and urinary retention are common Emergency Department (ED) presentations. The timely diagnosis of hydronephrosis in ureteric colic and ARF is valuable and may rapidly change management (e.g. prompting urgent decompression in pyonephrosis). Ultrasound (US) scanning of the kidneys and bladder is relatively easy to learn, particularly for emergency physicians who are trained in focused abdominal sonography in trauma (FAST).

Why use US?

- Bedside US is rapid, safe and does not require nephrotoxic contrast.
- US is sensitive in the diagnosis of hydronephrosis.
- US rapidly determines which patients with ARF require urgent intervention (e.g. nephrostomy).
- US confirms the diagnosis of urinary retention.
- US can be used to guide the safe placement of a suprapubic catheter (SPC).

Anatomy

Normal adult kidneys measure approximately 10–12 cm × 5 cm × 3 cm. Situated below the diaphragm, they lie obliquely in the retroperitoneum at the approximate level of vertebral bodies T12–L2. The right kidney lies more inferiorly than the left due to the bulk of the liver above (Fig. 11.1). Each kidney descends up to 2 cm in a full inspiration.

The kidney is invested in a capsule (brightly echogenic on US) surrounded by dark perinephric fat, which in turn is surrounded by fascia. The kidney may be divided into the renal cortex and medulla (dark on US) which surrounds the echogenic renal sinus, which consists of the pelvicalyceal system, renal vessels and fat (Figs 11.2 and 11.3). The calyces unite in the renal pelvis, which is the funnel-shaped origin of the ureter.

The bladder lies in the pelvis. As it fills it extends behind the symphysis pubis into the lower abdomen. A full bladder is dark (echo poor), well demarcated and demonstrates posterior acoustic enhancement.

103

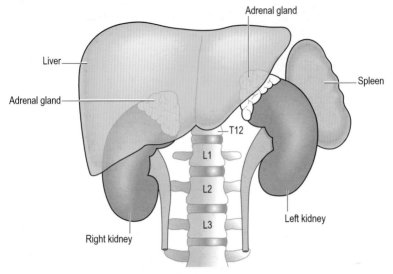

Fig. 11.1 *Anatomical relations of the kidneys, anterior view.*

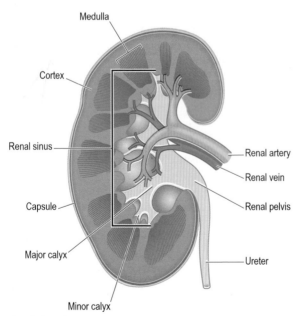

Fig. 11.2 *Kidney structure.*

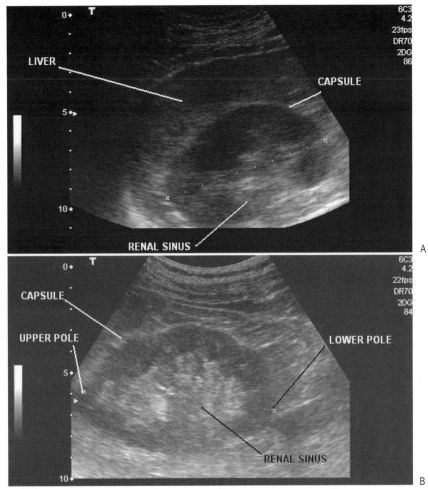

Fig. 11.3 *Longitudinal images of kidneys showing echogenic capsule, dark cortex and medulla, and bright renal sinus. Pole-to-pole measurement indicated. (A) Normal right kidney. (B) Normal left kidney.*

What US can tell you

Is the bladder full?

Acute urinary retention is commoner in elderly males with prostatic hypertrophy and is essentially a clinical diagnosis. However, clinical assessment of the bladder is difficult in some patients, for example the obese, and US can rapidly confirm the presence of a full bladder. It is also important to note that, in the presence of a distended bladder, hydronephrosis may be mimicked, i.e. a full bladder may lead to **false-positive** diagnosis of hydronephrosis.

Is there hydronephrosis?

Hydronephrosis may be defined as dilatation of the renal pelvis and calyces due to obstructed outflow of urine. For a diagnosis of hydronephrosis, the minimum anteroposterior (AP) diameter of the renal pelvis has been defined variously as 10 mm, 17 mm and 20 mm. This threshold also changes with age and pregnancy. For this reason, many radiologists prefer not to set an absolute threshold but to use a combination of findings (such as unilateral large kidney with renal pelvis and calyceal dilatation) to diagnose hydronephrosis.

Note that **calyceal dilatation** is also an important part of this definition, as the presence of pelvic dilatation with normal calyces may be found as a normal variant in patients with extrarenal pelvis.

Hydronephrosis is most commonly due to ureteric obstruction and may be acute or chronic. Acute hydronephrosis is of most interest to the ED physician in the following clinical situations:

- clinical presentation of renal colic and suspicion of ureteric calculus (stone)
- acute renal failure: to exclude post-renal cause (e.g. single kidney with obstructive uropathy).

What size are the kidneys?

In renal failure, the kidneys' dimensions and appearance on US will assist in formulating a differential diagnosis. For example, large, cystic kidneys suggest familial polycystic kidney disease. Bilaterally small, scarred kidneys suggest chronic renal disease such as long-standing glomerulonephritis. Significant difference in size between the kidneys suggests renovascular disease or reflux nephropathy.

Can I see a stone in the kidney or ureter?

On US a renal calculus is brightly echogenic and demonstrates posterior acoustic shadowing. A stone demonstrated in the renal pelvis (e.g. staghorn calculus) may be the cause of the patient's symptoms or incidental.

Where can I safely place the SPC?

As discussed below, US ensures adequate placement of the SPC.

What US can't tell you

- It cannot **exclude** a stone in the ureter. US is unable to image the ureters as they descend toward the bladder. Therefore it is poor at excluding ureteric calculi.
- It cannot determine the renal function. However the presence of small scarred kidneys suggests chronic renal failure.

The technique and views

Patient's position, probe and scanner settings

These are as for FAST (Ch. 4) with the patient supine. The decubitus position may be used (see below).

Probe placement and landmarks

1. *Right kidney.* Begin with probe parallel and between the ribs where the costal margin meets the mid axillary line on the right of the patient. Using the liver as an acoustic window, this view demonstrates right kidney, liver and highly echogenic diaphragm (Figs 4.6 and 4.7). The kidneys lie obliquely, so alter the probe angle until you obtain a clear long-axis view of the kidney. Ask the patient to take a deep breath if rib shadows obscure the kidney, to obtain a clearer view. Alter depth, focus and gain until the kidney image fills the screen.

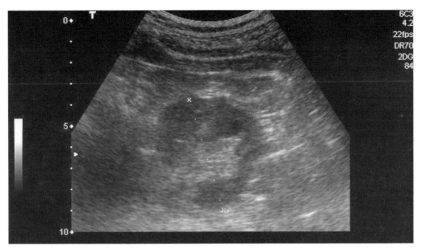

Fig. 11.4 *Right kidney transverse section with measurement.*

2. Measure the length of the kidney from pole to pole (Fig. 11.3), then rotate the probe to obtain a transverse or short-axis view and measure the dimensions (Fig. 11.4). For both axes, angle the probe back and forth to sweep the beam through as much of the kidney as possible.

3. *Left kidney.* This view is harder to obtain because the spleen is not as effective an acoustic window as the liver, and the kidney is higher. Begin on the left side as if looking for Morison's pouch but higher (ribs 9–11) and more posteriorly, in the posterior axillary line (Fig. 4.9). Again, a deep breath may help. Sweep the probe and alter its angle as above, until you obtain a clear view of left kidney, then alter depth and focus to improve the image.

4. An alternative method of scanning the left kidney is to lie the patient in the right decubitus position and scan through the left costovertebral angle (Fig. 11.5).

5. Another method is to place the probe in the right or left hypochondrium and direct it posteriorly. This view may be limited by bowel gas.

6. Hydronephrosis appears as a dark, echo-poor area in the pelvicalyceal system, communicating with the ureter (Fig. 11.6). Mild hydronephrosis may be subtle, but the presence of any dark, echo-poor areas within the normally bright renal sinus should raise the suspicion of hydronephrosis (Fig. 11.7).

7. Measure the anteroposterior (AP) diameter of the renal pelvis and compare the two kidneys. If one renal pelvis' diameter is greater than 10 mm, then hydronephrosis may be present (Fig. 11.8). (Note, however, that hydronephrosis may be bilateral.)

8. Assess the calyces. If they are also distended (Figs 11.6–11.8) then hydronephrosis is confirmed.

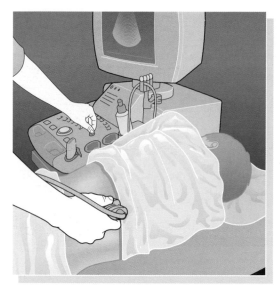

Fig. 11.5 *Patient in right decubitus position, probe scanning for left kidney.*

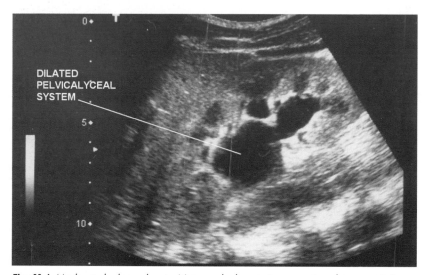

DILATED
PELVICALYCEAL
SYSTEM

Fig. 11.6 *Moderate hydronephrosis. Note marked posterior acoustic enhancement. For a better image, gain should be decreased deep to the fluid.*

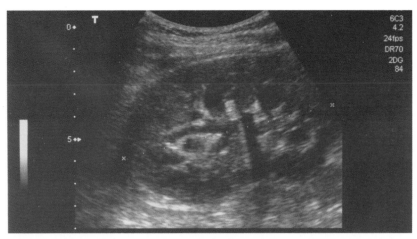

Fig. 11.7 *Mild hydronephrosis. Pelvic diameter has not been measured; however, calyces are dilated.*

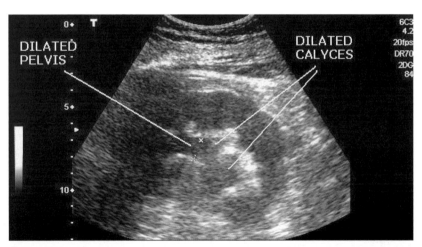

Fig. 11.8 *Hydronephrosis. Renal pelvis measures approximately 12.5 mm. Calyceal dilatation is also present and confirms the diagnosis.*

9. Chronic hydronephrosis is suggested by thinning of the renal cortex.
10. Cysts may mimic hydronephrosis. They are also echo-poor but are found in the cortex rather than the collecting system and do not communicate with the renal pelvis (Fig. 11.9). Cysts are a common finding and may be benign or malignant. The presence of multiple cysts suggests polycystic kidney disease (PCKD) or age-related multicystic disease (Fig. 11.10).

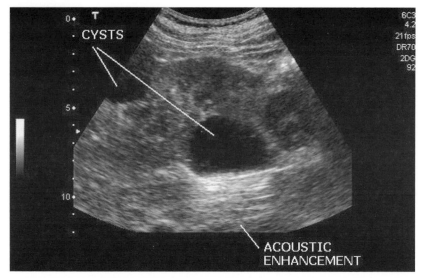

Fig. 11.9 Renal cysts. Note posterior acoustic enhancement behind large cyst.

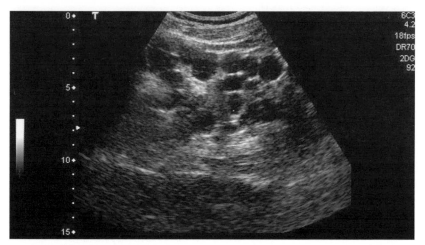

Fig. 11.10 Multiple renal cysts.

11. When seen on US, calculi are brightly echogenic and demonstrate posterior acoustic shadowing.
12. *Bladder.* Scan as for FAST (Ch. 4), with the probe angled into the pelvis.

Suprapubic catheterization

This is used in the patient in acute retention in whom urethral catheterization is difficult or contraindicated. This may be performed using real-time US guidance (described below) or the site identified using US prior to insertion of a suprapubic catheter (SPC).

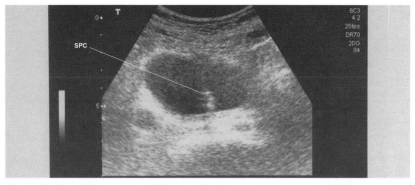

Fig. 11.11 *Suprapubic catheter (SPC) tip in bladder.*

1. Informed consent, dedicated suprapubic catheter (SPC), local anaesthetic, sterile equipment and sterile US sheath as per local practice.
2. Using US, confirm full bladder as above and identify a site in the midline above the symphysis pubis with no structures overlying the bladder. Mark the site and clean the skin using full aseptic technique.
3. Administer local anaesthetic. While the anaesthetic is taking effect, place the probe inside a sterile sheath and image the bladder again, confirming the optimal site for SPC insertion.
4. Incise the skin with a scalpel to aid SPC passage.
5. Introduce the SPC and introducer, monitoring progress into the bladder (Fig. 11.11).
6. Observe 'flashback' of urine, remove introducer and secure SPC following manufacturer's instructions.

Positives and negatives

- Left kidney, normal longitudinal section (Fig. 11.3)
- Right kidney, normal transverse section (Fig. 11.4)
- Hydronephrosis (Figs 11.6, 11.7 and 11.8)
- Renal cysts (Figs 11.9 and 11.10).

Handy hints and caveats

✔ Avoid misdiagnosis of 'ureteric colic' in patients with more sinister pathology such as symptomatic abdominal aortic aneurysm (see Ch. 3: AAA).

✔ The left kidney is more posterior and more cranial than you think!

✔ Scan through the respiratory cycle to minimize the effects of rib shadowing.

✔ If available, a probe with a particularly small footprint can scan between ribs.

✔ If you still find it difficult to identify the kidneys, slide the probe proximally until you view the highly echogenic diaphragm. Use this as a landmark and slide the probe distally.

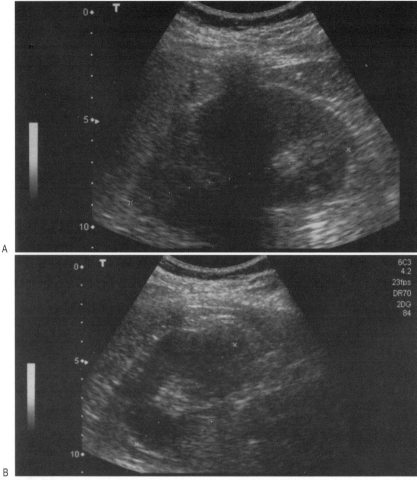

Fig. 11.12 (A) Accurate measurement of kidney length. Both poles are seen. (B) Inaccurate estimation: plane of probe is oblique to long axis of kidney.

✔ If a kidney is still not visible or displays unusual features, consider congenital abnormalities such as absent or horseshoe kidney.

✔ Scanning a transplanted kidney (usually found in the iliac fossa) is usually easier as the kidney is more superficial than native kidneys.

✔ When measuring kidney dimensions, avoid underestimation of length, which can occur if the US beam intersects the kidney obliquely or if both poles are not seen simultaneously (Fig. 11.12).

✔ Remember to compare the left and right kidneys (e.g. when assessing renal dimensions).

✔ Beware **false positives** for hydronephrosis. These may be found in pregnant patients, those with extrarenal pelvis (a normal variant) and normal patients with a distended bladder.

✔ Beware **false negatives**. Hydronephrosis may not be obvious if early or in a dehydrated patient. The presence of any dark, echo-poor areas within the normally bright renal sinus should raise the suspicion of hydronephrosis.

✔ If the renal pelvis **and calyces** are dilated, then hydronephrosis is present.

✔ If inserting a suprapubic catheter, either prior US site identification or real-time US guidance may be used.

Now what?

• Hydronephrosis in a patient with single kidney and ARF: urgent decompression (e.g. nephrostomy) by the radiologists or urologists.

• Clinical and US features of pyonephrosis also mandate urgent decompression.

• Clinical picture of ureteric colic plus hydronephrosis strongly suggests the presence of ureteric calculus. Assess for severity (e.g. mild versus gross hydronephrosis) and complications (such as infection and renal impairment) and discuss with urologists.

• Clinical picture of ureteric colic, **no** hydronephrosis: arrange further imaging for ureteric calculus (e.g. non-contrast CT) as per local protocol.

• Clinical picture of urinary retention, distended bladder on US: proceed to urethral or suprapubic catheterization.

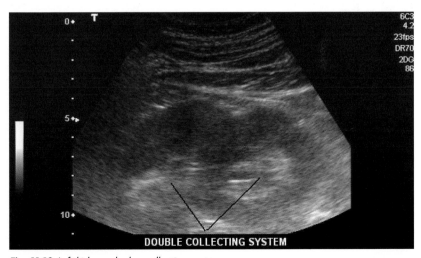

DOUBLE COLLECTING SYSTEM

Fig. 11.13 *Left kidney, duplex collecting system.*

- Inadequate scan, other pathology (e.g. multiple cysts, duplex collecting system (Fig 11.13), bladder wall thickening or mass) or other question (e.g. are there urinary flow jets visible in the bladder?): arrange further imaging, for example CT or formal US.

 Avoid misdiagnosis of 'ureteric colic' in patients with more sinister pathology such as symptomatic abdominal aortic aneurysm (AAA).

Summary

→ US scanning of the kidneys and bladder is rapid and easy to learn.
→ US confirmation of hydronephrosis requires demonstration of:
  → renal pelvis dilatation
  → associated calyceal dilatation.
→ Inability to view the kidneys adequately should prompt the clinician to arrange formal US.
→ Other disease entities (such as symptomatic AAA) must also be considered in patients with presumptive diagnosis of ureteric colic.

Chapter 12

Gallbladder

Justin Bowra

Introduction

Gallstone disease is common and is responsible for a range of emergency presentations. US scanning of the gallbladder (GB) is relatively easy to learn, particularly for emergency physicians who are trained in FAST.

Why use US?

- US is sensitive in the detection of stones in the GB.
- US is sensitive in the diagnosis of acute cholecystitis.

Anatomy

Gallbladder. The GB has a capacity of about 50 ml. It lies in the GB fossa below the liver, between the liver's right and quadrate lobes. It may be divided into neck, body and fundus.

The GB fundus projects below the liver (surface marking: intersection of costal margin and lateral border right rectus sheath). However, the exact position and shape of the fundus varies with its volume, patient anatomy and fasting status (Fig. 12.1). The GB body is the continuation of the fundus and narrows towards the neck, which continues into the cystic duct.

Biliary tree. The cystic duct is 2–3 cm long and has a normal diameter of 2 mm or less. It joins the common hepatic duct (formed by the union of the right and left hepatic ducts) to form the common bile duct (CBD). The CBD descends in the hepatoduodenal ligament with the portal vein and the hepatic artery. It joins the pancreatic duct at the ampulla of Vater, which opens into the duodenum.

What emergency US can tell you

- Is there a stone in the GB?
- Is the GB inflamed? **Acute cholecystitis** usually is caused by gallstone impaction of the GB neck or cystic duct. Diagnosis requires a **combination** of the following, as each individual finding may be found in other disease states:
  - clinical features, e.g. fever and right upper quadrant pain and tenderness
  - sonographic Murphy's sign (see below)
  - impacted gallstone: present in most cases, but may be difficult to view if in the cystic duct. Acalculous cholecystitis is rare but carries a worse prognosis

115

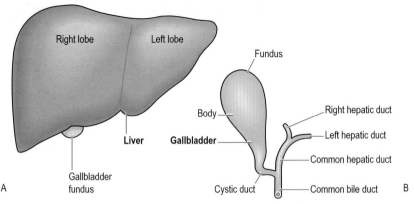

A

B

Fig. 12.1 *Gallbladder anatomy. (A) Anterior aspect: gallbladder fundus projecting below liver. (B) Gallbladder and extrahepatic biliary tree.*

* GB wall thickening
* pericholecystic fluid.

What emergency US can't tell you

* Can I **exclude** a stone in the GB? Several views are required to completely exclude small GB calculi. However, small asymptomatic stones are of little clinical concern to the ED clinician.
* Other pathology, such as biliary dilatation. Emergency US is not a substitute for a formal hepatobiliary US. For example, because the bile ducts are tubular structures and are found with blood vessels, which they may resemble (e.g. the CBD may be mistaken for either the portal vein or hepatic artery), experience and Doppler are required for confident identification of the bile ducts. Hence, if you are concerned about the possibility of biliary dilatation or other pathology (such as tumours), arrange formal US.

 Formal upper abdominal US is complex and includes assessment of the hepatobiliary system, pancreas and other structures. Hence, it requires equipment and experience not possessed by ED sonographers.

The technique and views

Patient's position, probe and scanner settings

* As for FAST (Ch. 4).
* Supine position is most practical in the unwell patient.
* An alternative is left lateral decubitus, as for cardiac scanning (Fig. 10.1, Shock and arrest). In this position, a poorly visualized GB may drop into view.
* Alternative patient positions (such as right lateral, decubitus and even erect) are sometimes required for a complete view of the GB.

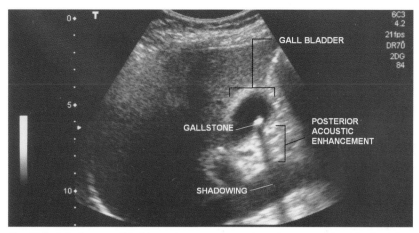

Fig. 12.2 Calculus in gallbladder with posterior acoustic enhancement from fluid, and posterior acoustic shadowing from stone.

• Fasting status: the GB contracts with meals and therefore may be harder to view if the patient has recently eaten.

Probe placement and landmarks

1. Commence with the probe aligned longitudinally in the mid-axillary line, at the costal margin or just subcostal (as for FAST).

2. Identify the landmarks: right kidney, liver and diaphragm (highly echogenic) (Fig. 4.7). Scan through the phases of respiration to assist visualization of the GB.

3. The fasted GB appears as a well-demarcated fluid-filled structure inferior to the liver (Figs 2.9 and 12.2). Alter depth and focus settings to maximise your view of the GB. Scan through the GB by altering probe angle and position and attempt to obtain longitudinal and transverse views of the GB.

4. Is this the GB? Confirm that the fluid-filled structure is indeed the GB (and not a loop of bowel) by scanning in two planes and by demonstrating the GB neck narrowing toward the cystic duct, or by the presence of calculi.

5. GB calculi appear as highly reflective echoes with posterior acoustic shadows (Figs 12.2 and 12.3). Echoes which do not cast shadows usually represent sludging.

6. To diagnose an **impacted** gallstone, scan the patient in more than one position (e.g. decubitus). An impacted gallstone does not move with gravity.

7. Sonographic Murphy's sign: place the probe in the right upper quadrant of the abdomen, **under** the costal margin, angled upwards (Fig. 12.4). If a patient's abdominal pain is reproduced with probe pressure over the GB, this strongly suggests GB disease as the cause of the patient's symptoms.

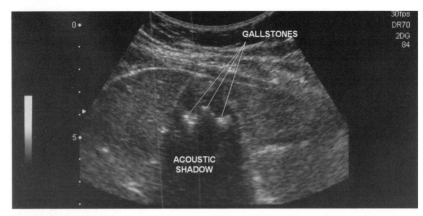

Fig. 12.3 Multiple gallstones.

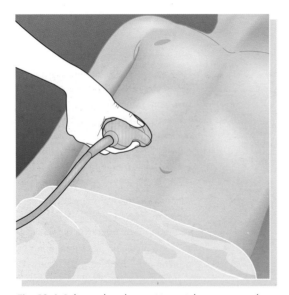

Fig. 12.4 Subcostal probe position, right upper quadrant, probe angled upwards.

8. The subcostal position just described may yield a useful alternative view of the GB.
9. GB wall:
   - Thickness: normal adult wall thickness is 3 mm or less. A thickened wall usually appears as two echogenic lines with a hypoechoic region between them (Figs 12.5 and 12.6). This suggests acute inflammation but may also be found in other disease states (e.g. congestive cardiac failure and sepsis). In addition, normal non-fasted GB walls will also be thickened due to contraction. This is important to remember in the non-fasted ED population.

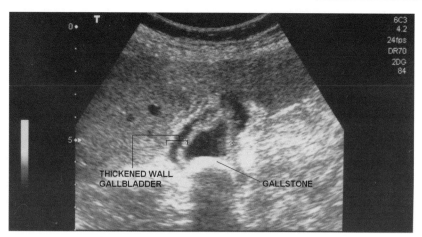

Fig. 12.5 *Acute cholecystitis and impacted stone, transverse section. Gallbladder wall thickening with localized free fluid.*

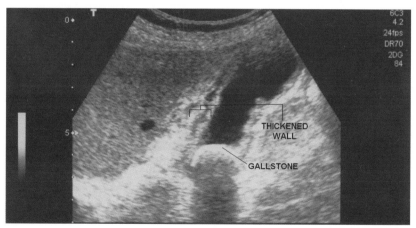

Fig. 12.6 *Same patient as in Fig. 12.5, longitudinal section gallbladder. Note that the gallstone's posterior shadowing in both images is less obvious because of concomitant acoustic enhancement due to fluid and liver. Solution: decrease gain.*

- Other wall findings, e.g. focal wall thickening (e.g. carcinoma) or calcification, can be found in a variety of diseases which are beyond the scope of this book.

10. Air in the GB lumen or wall: emphysematous cholecystitis is a rare surgical emergency. Air in the lumen is usually hyper-echoic but without posterior shadowing. Air in the walls may simulate calcification.

119

11. Free fluid (FF) around the GB: localized fluid around the GB is usually found in acute cholecystitis (particularly with GB perforation) but may be found in other disease states such as pancreatitis.

Positives and negatives

* GB with gallstone (Fig. 12.2)
* GB, multiple gallstones (Fig. 12.3)
* GB, acute cholecystitis (Figs 12.5 and 12.6)

Handy hints and caveats

✔ The GB is most easily seen in the fasted patient. Beware physiological GB wall thickening in the non-fasted patient.

✔ Congenital variations (such as duplication) are rare.

✔ More than one window, scanning plane and patient position may be required to view the GB.

✔ If possible, a deep inspiration will improve your view.

✔ In itself, the presence of stones does not infer cholecystitis. Asymptomatic stones are a common incidental finding.

✔ Similarly, GB wall thickening alone may be found in other disease states besides acute cholecystitis.

✔ An impacted stone in the **cystic duct** may be difficult for the ED sonographer to detect. Therefore, if the other clinical and sonographic features of acute cholecystitis are present, the diagnosis may be inferred.

✔ Inability to view the GB, or abnormal findings such as focal wall thickening or calcification should prompt the clinician to arrange formal radiological investigation such as US or CT.

✔ Occasionally a GB becomes completely filled with gallstones. When this occurs, the normal fluid-filled structure with posterior enhancement is no longer seen. Instead, two parallel bright lines with posterior shadowing are seen. This represents **wall-echo shadow (WES)**. The bright line nearer the probe is the GB wall. The line beneath represents the echogenic stone. In multiple stones this second line is often irregular. WES is important because it may be misinterpreted as a bowel loop but in fact represents cholelithiasis.

Diagnosis of acute cholecystitis requires a combination of clinical signs (e.g. sonographic Murphy's sign) and US findings (e.g. calculi, GB wall thickening and pericholecystic fluid).

Gallstones are a common incidental finding. In isolation, their presence does not infer cholecystitis or biliary colic.

Now what?

- Acute cholecystitis: consult surgeons immediately.
- Clinical picture of biliary colic, gallstones demonstrated: discuss with surgeons.
- No features of GB disease, sonographic Murphy's negative: seek other cause of patient's symptoms.
- Inadequate scan, more complex pathology sought or clinical picture of biliary disease and unable to detect gallstones: arrange formal US.

Summary

→ US scanning of the GB is rapid and easy to learn.
→ US is sensitive in the detection of GB calculi and acute cholecystitis.
→ Emergency US is not a substitute for formal sonography.
→ Inability to view the GB, or abnormal findings such as focal wall thickening or calcification should prompt the clinician to arrange formal US.

Chapter 13

Early pregnancy

Sabrina Kuah, Justin Bowra, Tony Joseph

Introduction

The symptoms of an ectopic pregnancy (EP) (e.g. abdominal pain, amenorrhoea and vaginal bleeding in a patient with a positive pregnancy test) can be difficult to distinguish from other complications of early pregnancy such as spontaneous abortion, ruptured corpus luteum cyst or unrelated illness such as acute appendicitis. Likewise, examination may prove unremarkable, especially with an early unruptured EP. Ultrasound (US) is non-invasive and can be performed with little delay (during resuscitation of the patient if necessary) and correlated with a quantitative serum beta-human chorionic gonadotropin (βHCG). Serial US and βHCG are essential for monitoring equivocal cases.

The question: is there an ectopic pregnancy?

An EP can be defined as a pregnancy outside the uterine cavity. Its incidence varies geographically from 1 in 28 to 1 in 300 pregnancies (19 per 1000 pregnancies in USA), with 65% occurring in the age group 25–34 years. Some 98% of EPs occur in the fallopian tube, with the remainder being abdominal, ovarian or cervical.

Despite early detection due to transvaginal ultrasound (TVS) and βHCG, EP remains the leading cause of pregnancy-related maternal death in the first trimester, accounting for about 10% of all pregnancy-related deaths.

Risk factors for EP include previous EP (odds ratio 8.3), tubal pathology (OR 3.5–25) and previous tubal surgery (OR 21).

Some 2–3% of EPs may be interstitial. In these cases the EP is located in the interstitial part of the fallopian tube as it traverses the uterine wall and the main part of the gestational sac is located **outside** the uterine cavity. The mortality of these pregnancies is twice that of other tubal pregnancies (2%) as they tend to rupture later (at 8–16 weeks' gestation).

Heterotopic pregnancy (defined as co-existing intrauterine and extrauterine pregnancy) is rare: 1 in 30 000 spontaneous conceptions and 1:100 to 1:3000 technically assisted conceptions.

Why use US?

Bedside US is safe and can be performed at the bedside without interrupting patient resuscitation. Two methods are used: transabdominal (TA) and transvaginal (TV). The TV method is more accurate and achieves better resolution of pelvic structures (Figs 13.1–13.3). Unlike TA scanning, it does not require a full bladder. However, TV scanning is invasive and requires more exhaustive training than TA and consequently is outside the scope of this text.

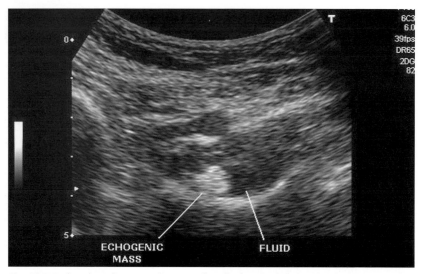

Fig. 13.1 *Right adnexal mass with surrounding fluid, transabdominal (TA) scan. 6 weeks gestational age (GA), βHCG >1000 and pseudosac in uterus. Formal US (including transvaginal, TV) confirmed right adnexal ectopic pregnancy (EP). Scan lacks the resolution of the TV scans which follow.*

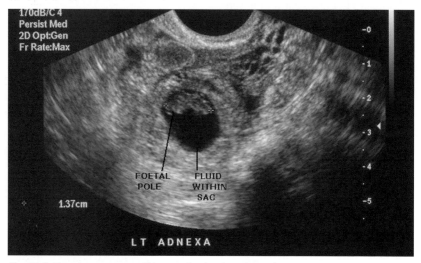

Fig. 13.2 *Ectopic pregnancy, TV scan. Fetal pole indicated.*

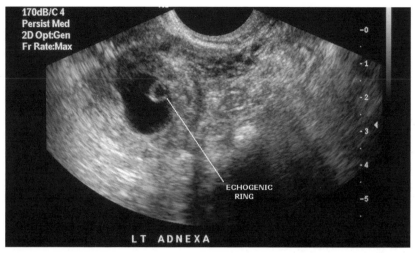

170dB/C 4
Persist Med
2D Opt:Gen
Fr Rate:Max

ECHOGENIC
RING

LT ADNEXA

Fig. 13.3 *Ectopic pregnancy, TV scan. Echogenic ring indicated.*

One advantage of TA over TV scanning is its ability to assess the abdomen and upper pelvis. Pathology here may be missed on a TV scan, because the higher-frequency transducer limits the depth of view to the lower pelvis.

A TA scan performed by an emergency physician does not seek to replace a formal ultrasound study. It is an on-the-spot tool to assist in the assessment of early pregnancy. For example, it may be used to identify patients with a definite *in utero* pregnancy (IUP). Given the rare incidence of heterotopic pregnancy, a stable uncomplicated patient with a live IUP demonstrated on ultrasound is a good candidate for discharge with appropriate follow up.

Conversely, all patients with an equivocal ultrasound (i.e. one in which a definite IUP is not identified) require a gynaecological (OG) consultation.

Studies (Mateer et al 1996, Shih 1997) indicate that ultrasound-trained ED physicians can reliably determine the presence of an IUP. Shih demonstrated that screening ultrasounds performed in this context decreased ED stay by almost 120 minutes. Mateer et al demonstrated a significant decrease in morbidity secondary to missed EP when an ultrasound-trained ED physician performed a screening ultrasound prior to selecting patients appropriate for discharge from the ED.

What emergency US can tell you

- Is there an EP? Most EPs will **not** demonstrate an extrauterine gestational sac containing a yolk sac or embryo. However, the finding of an adnexal mass in a patient with an empty uterus and elevated βHCG makes EP likely.
- Is there free fluid (FF)? US can detect the presence of FF in the Pouch of Douglas, which may be due to a bleeding EP or a haemorrhagic/ ruptured cyst.

Table 13.1 Transabdominal (TA) findings in normal pregnancy. Note that the timings indicated below are estimates only and vary with patient habitus, machine quality and operator skill. All findings below will appear earlier with TV scanning. Note also that gestational age calculations based on last menstrual period (LMP) can be wrong!

Approx. 5 weeks, βHCG >1800	Gestational sac (including yolk sac). Yolk sac should be seen by 7 weeks in normal IUP
7 weeks	Fetal pole (should be visible when mean gestational sac measurement is >25 mm). Embryo should be seen by 8 weeks
7 weeks	Fetal cardiac activity (note: if you can see fetal pole on TA scan you should always be able to detect cardiac activity)

IUP = *in utero* pregnancy.

- Is there an IUP? Except in the rare incidence of heterotopic pregnancy (beware assisted reproduction treatment patients), identification of an IUP practically excludes EP.
- Is the uterus empty? An empty uterus in a woman with a positive pregnancy test is highly suggestive of an EP.

What emergency US can't tell you

- Is the IUP normal? Leave comments such as 'normal pregnancy' to the formal sonographers. However, the presence of a true gestational sac, fetal pole and fetal heart beat are reassuring features.
- If I demonstrate an IUP, can I rule out an EP completely? Not always. For example, an **interstitial** pregnancy can be difficult to distinguish from an IUP that is eccentrically placed—look for a gestational sac or hyperechoic mass in the cornua with myometrial thinning. A hyper-echoic 'interstitial line' may be seen extending from the uterine cavity to the cornual gestational sac. If in doubt, arrange formal US.

The role of βHCG

Of all the laboratory parameters which may discriminate between a viable IUP and an EP, βHCG is the most useful. In the presence of a pregnancy, βHCG can be detected prior to a missed menses and can remain elevated for weeks after pregnancy demise.

When assessing serum βHCG, it is important to consider:

- **The absolute level.** Most viable IUPs will be visible on TVS at a βHCG level of >1500 IU/L and TA scan at a βHCG >1800. Hence, if TA scan demonstrates an empty uterus and βHCG >1800, suspect EP. However, a level below 1500 must not be interpreted as 'no EP' or 'no risk of EP rupture'.

 βHCG <1500 does not rule out EP.

- *Whether the βHCG is rising or falling.* For example, in the case above (βHCG >1500, empty uterus), if this is a wanted pregnancy in a stable patient, the OG team may elect to repeat the βHCG and TVS in 2 days. A falling βHCG is consistent with a failed pregnancy (non-viable IUP, tubal abortion, spontaneously resolving EP).
- *The rate of decline.* βHCG falls **more slowly** with an EP than with a completed abortion. Hence, if the βHCG falls by more than 50% in 48 hours in the presence of an indeterminate US, an EP is very unlikely and most likely there is a spontaneous abortion.
- *The rate of rise.* Some 85% of viable IUPs demonstrate a mean doubling time of 1.4 to 2.1 days until day 40 when βHCG reaches a plateau of 100 000. While this can also be said for a minority of EPs, the rise in βHCG in most patients with EP is much slower. Hence, if the βHCG is **failing to double** over 72 hours and repeat TVS shows an empty uterus, the pregnancy is non-viable regardless of location and treatment for EP can be initiated as appropriate. Conversely, a normal rise in βHCG needs to be monitored with serial TVS until the location of the gestation can be visualized.

Clinical picture

- The patient: female and fertile.
- Pregnancy: always assume a woman of child-bearing age is pregnant and test serum βHCG.
- Classic features such as pain, shock and vaginal bleeding may not be present.

 If in doubt, assume that the patient has EP until proven otherwise.

Before you scan

- Initial resuscitation as clinically indicated.
- Get help: the doctor performing the scan should not also be resuscitating the patient.
- If the patient is unstable, contact OG before you scan.
- Send blood for full blood count, quantitative βHCG and either group and hold or cross match as indicated.

The technique and views: TA scan

Patient's position

- Supine is most practical.
- Full bladder if possible. (It is possible to perform TA scan without a full bladder if you do not have time to allow the bladder to fill, but the results will be much harder to interpret. Consider referral for TV scan or urgent OG review in such situations.)
- A bimanual pelvic examination prior to an ultrasound examination may be helpful—e.g. localization of a mass or tenderness may direct a TA scan.

Probe and scanner settings

- Curved probe: suggested frequency 2.5–5 MHz.
- Begin with standard B-mode setting.
- If available, M-mode also should be used to demonstrate the fetal heart beat.
- Standard orientation: patient's right is on *left* of screen.
- Adjust image depth and focus according to the patient's habitus.

127

Probe placement and landmarks

- Commence with the probe in the midline just above the pubis (Figs 4.12 and 4.15). Identify the bladder (as in Ch. 4: *FAST*). Use the full bladder as a sonographic 'window' to deeper structures.

- Scanning transversely and longitudinally, identify the uterus as it lies behind the bladder, documenting its size, shape and orientation (Fig. 13.4). Alter image depth and focus as required. In pregnancy, the uterus appears as a thick-walled, hollow muscular structure with non-echogenic fluid. The normal non-pregnant uterus in a woman of child-bearing age is less than 10 cm long and less than 6 cm in width. Identify the myometrium, endometrium (which appears as a thin, hyperechoic line) and cervix.

- Focus on the uterine cavity: scan longitudinally and transversely through the cavity for evidence of an IUP—an intrauterine gestational sac with a yolk sac, fetal pole or cardiac motion (M-mode). (See below for details.)

- Then identify the two ovaries, which appear oval and hypo-echoic. Ideally, one should document their volume in millilitres (mL). However, the details of ovarian volume measurement are beyond the scope of this text.

- Unlike the ovaries, fallopian tubes are not usually visible unless dilated.

- The adnexae are not seen as a specific structure on transabdominal US.

- Evaluate the cul-de-sac for free fluid, echogenic rings and masses.

- Use gentle probe pressure and angling to differentiate any pathological structure (such as a ring or mass) from ovarian pathology such as a ruptured corpus luteum. Identify whether any pathological structure moves independently of the ovary. (Often this is easier to demonstrate transvaginally.)

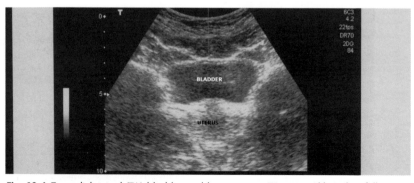

Fig. 13.4 *Transabdominal (TA) bladder and lower uterus, TA scan. Although a full bladder assists visualization of the uterus, care must be taken to ensure that posterior acoustic enhancement does not render deeper structures too bright, as in this case. Solution: decrease the gain.*

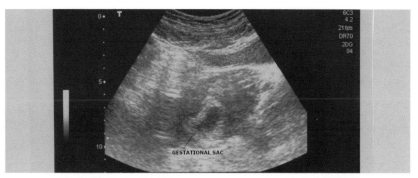

GESTATIONAL SAC

Fig. 13.5 *Gestational sac but no yolk sac, TA scan. 6 weeks gestational age (GA). Patient referred for formal US, which demonstrated yolk sac.*

- Finally, methodically sweep through the lower abdomen and pelvis. Pathology here may be missed by TV scans, which concentrate on the lower pelvis.
- Similarly, a modified FAST (see Ch. 4) may identify free fluid elsewhere in the abdomen.

Essential views and findings

1. Normal IUP: this usually excludes EP (except in the rare circumstance of heterotopic pregnancy). A normal IUP should demonstrate the following:
   - The true gestational sac (Fig. 13.5) is the first true sign of pregnancy on US and represents the chorionic cavity (sac itself), implanting chorionic villi and associated decidual tissue (outer echogenic region). Initially it appears as an echogenic ring, representing a small fluid-filled sac embedded below the midline. As it enlarges, it becomes more elliptical. Initially there is nothing distinctive visible in the sac cavity. Hence, it may be confused with a pseudosac (see below).

- The mean sac diameter (MSD) is the average measurement of the sac (excluding the echogenic rim) in three planes. By measuring the MSD of a very early pregnancy, the gestational age (GA) can be calculated by referring to a chart or applying this rule of thumb: **30 + MSD in mm = GA in days.** As the pregnancy progresses the MSD increases by 1 mm/day while the outer echogenic region remains the same (2 mm or more).
- The spherical **yolk sac** should be taken as the first **definite** sign of pregnancy on US. It is the first anatomical structure seen inside a gestational sac and may be seen from an MSD of 5 mm, although it may not appear until MSD 8 mm. When first visible on US it is a perfect echogenic ring inside the gestational sac. This combination of a hyperechoic 'ring' (the yolk sac) within the hyperechoic outer gestational sac is known as the **'double decidual sac'** sign (Fig. 13.6).

129

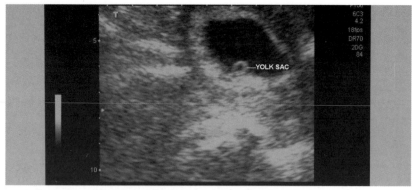

Fig. 13.6 *Yolk sac, transabdominal (TA) scan.*

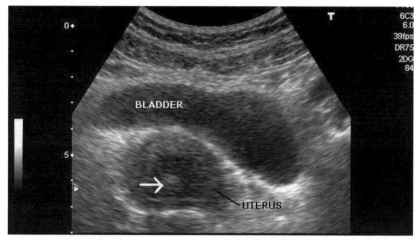

Fig. 13.7 *Pseudosac, TA scan. Same patient as in Fig. 13.1. Fluid-filled sac within uterus contains echogenic debris which may be mistaken for a fetal pole (arrowed).*

- By contrast, the **pseudosac** (pseudogestational sac) has only a single hyper-echoic layer, no yolk sac 'ring' within it, no fetal pole and no cardiac activity. It is seen in 10–20% of EPs due to the hormonal changes in pregnancy and may display a low-level echo pattern due to debris in its cavity, particularly in patients with a high level of βHCG (Fig. 13.7).

- At 6 weeks the embryonic disc (thickened region at the edge of the yolk sac) may be visible with the fetal pole and cardiac activity (M-mode) detectable from 7 weeks (Fig. 13.8).
- Eventually the fetus begins to have a recognizable appearance (Fig. 13.9).

- The yolk sac continues to grow to a maximum diameter of 6 mm by 10 weeks, all the while migrating to the periphery until it is no longer visible by the end of the first trimester.

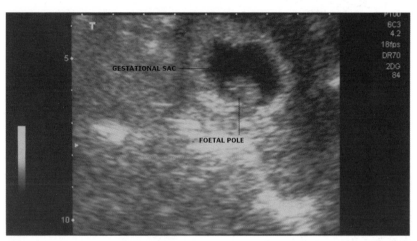

Fig. 13.8 *Fetal pole, TA scan. 8 weeks gestational age (GA). M-mode scan demonstrated fetal heartbeat.*

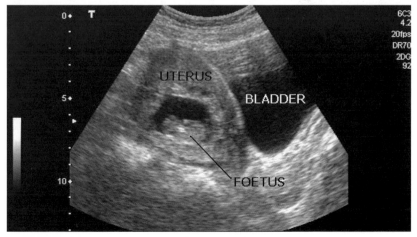

Fig. 13.9 *Fetal parts, TA scan. Ten weeks gestational age (GA).*

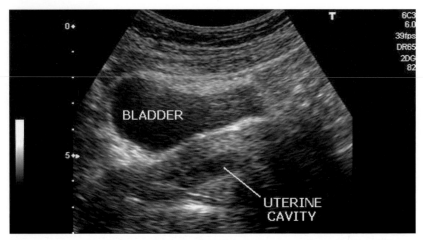

Fig. 13.10 *Empty uterus longitudinal section, TA scan. Gestational age (GA) 6 weeks, positive pregnancy test. TV scan demonstrated ectopic pregnancy (EP).*

- Fetal heartbeat. This may be visible as a rapid 'flicker' within the fetal pole. If M-mode is available, direct the scanning line through the fetal pole to demonstrate cardiac activity.

2. US findings in ectopic pregnancy:

- An embryo with cardiac activity outside the uterus is diagnostic but is found in only 8–26% of EPs (Fig. 13.2).
- More commonly (40–70%) an 'echogenic ring' is visualized outside the uterus (Fig. 13.3).
- The combination of an echogenic adnexal mass, an empty uterus and a positive pregnancy test carries 85% likelihood of EP.
- A ruptured EP may appear as a complex adnexal mass of mixed echogenicity.
- An **empty uterus** alone (or pseudogestational sac) is suggestive of EP but may represent other states such as miscarriage or even early normal IUP (Fig. 13.10).

- Intraperitoneal haemorrhage can result in cul-de-sac fluid, which may be particulate depending on its age. The combination of positive pregnancy test, free fluid and an empty uterus carries a 71% risk of EP. This rises to 95% if a large amount of free fluid is present.
- The combination of an echogenic mass and free fluid makes EP almost certain.
- An ovarian EP can be difficult to distinguish from a haemorrhagic corpus luteum or corpus luteum cyst as both will move with the ovary. If available, colour Doppler demonstrates a 'ring of fire' around the highly vascular, usually viable trophoblastic tissue of an EP. However, to a lesser extent a corpus luteum may have a similar appearance.

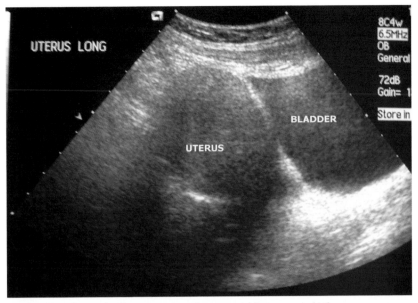

Fig. 13.11 *TA longitudinal scan uterus, indeterminate. Gain set too high.*

- Interstitial EPs are richly vascular and can remain viable for some time, growing to a large size. Initially appearing as an asymmetrical IUP, the cornual ectopic is not actually within the uterine cavity. Look for a hyperechoic 'interstitial line' extending from the uterine cavity to the cornual gestational sac.
- Likewise a cervical EP is not in the uterine cavity (differential diagnosis: imminent miscarriage).
- Some 20–30% of EPs have no detectable sonographic abnormalities at the time of diagnosis.

Positives and negatives

- IUP with gestational sac but yolk sac not identified, TA scan (Fig. 13.5).
- IUP with yolk sac, TA scan (Fig. 13.6).
- IUP with fetal pole, TA scan (Fig. 13.8).

- IUP with fetal parts, TA scan (Fig. 13.9).
- Empty uterus, positive pregnancy test (Fig. 13.10).
- EP, TA scan (Fig. 13.1).
- Indeterminate TA scans (Figs 13.11 and 13.12).

Handy hints

- ✔ If in doubt, assume that the patient has EP until proven otherwise.
- ✔ Urgently refer all shocked patients with suspected EP to the gynaecologists. Do not waste time performing a TA scan before referral.
- ✔ You are not a sonographer! Refer all indeterminate scans for formal US or urgent OG review, as dictated by clinical picture.
- ✔ A full bladder is required for best results in a TA scan. If empty, either push fluids or refer for TV scan.
- ✔ βHCG <1500 does not rule out EP.

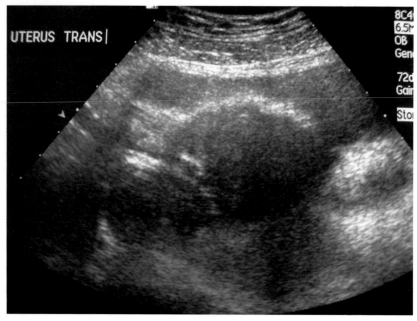

Fig. 13.12 *TA transverse scan uterus, indeterminate.*

✔ Hence if EP is suspected as a possibility, it is reasonable to perform a US regardless of βHCG level.

✔ Due to inter-assay variability (10–15% variability) serial monitoring should take place in the same laboratory.

✔ If using M-mode function, **do not use pulsed Doppler**. This may adversely affect the fetus. Refer to your machine's operation manual or discuss with local radiologist or sonographer.

✔ False positives for EP:
   ✔ early normal IUP (prior to appearance of yolk sac)
   ✔ miscarriage
   ✔ corpus luteum cyst.

✔ False negatives for EP:
   ✔ intrauterine pseudosac
   ✔ interstitial EP
   ✔ heterotopic pregnancy (extremely rare); such patients usually have had assisted reproduction.

 Beware the pseudosac!

Now what?

• Unstable patient: resuscitate and notify OG immediately.
   • If EP is suspected or identified, the patient must be transferred immediately to OT.
   • If unable to rule out EP, decision to proceed to OT (or further imaging) must be based on clinical likelihood of EP.

• Stable patient, IUP confirmed, no RF for heterotopia: EP effectively has been ruled out. Refer for outpatient OG review.

• Stable patient, IUP confirmed, but patient has RF for heterotopia: further assessment as for EP.

- Stable patient, βHCG >1800, empty uterus and/or other suspicious findings such as adnexal mass on TA scan: suspect EP and notify OG.
- Stable patient, βHCG <1800, empty uterus: this is a complex situation and must be discussed with OG. TV scan should be performed by OG. If TV scan is also negative, local practices will differ. Options include monitoring the patient and repeating βHCG and TVS in 2–3 days.

 If in doubt, assume that the patient has EP until proven otherwise.

Summary

TA scanning by ED physicians is not a substitute for formal US. However, in conjunction with serum βHCG it is an invaluable tool in the ED to assist diagnosis of abdominal pain or vaginal bleeding in the first trimester.

Chapter 14

Getting trained and staying trained

Russell McLaughlin, Fergal Cummins

Introduction: educational principles

There are two distinct areas to be considered when a practitioner chooses to engage in ultrasound (US) training:

1. Psychomotor skills. This is the actual process of doing the scan. It begins with switching the machine on and finishes with the production of an image. This is a technical skill and can be learned by observing an expert deconstruct the process into small steps followed by the student reconstructing the process. These are the same principles that are used to teach practical skills on many of the recognized resuscitation and trauma courses. Radiographer-ultrasonographers represent an excellent resource in this area.
2. Deductive reasoning. This is the hard part. It is the process of:
   - viewing an image in conjunction with a clinical picture
   - formulating a hypothesis as to a differential diagnosis.

This draws upon a huge range of medical knowledge, skills and experience. Educationalists have demonstrated that this process cannot be learned in the same way as psychomotor skills. To enhance deductive reasoning requires a structured learning programme tailored to the individual's needs.

Types of course

The emergency US courses available to clinicians fall into two broad categories:

- An introductory or basic course, which focuses on the core basic knowledge, principles and skills of US with goal-directed aims
- An advanced course directed towards a broader clinical usage of US.

Currently there is no national or international standardization of core course content.

Introductory emergency US course

A typical introductory course is held over a 1- or 2-day period. It consists of a combination of traditional lecturing sections and plenty of 'hands on' practical sessions. The practical sessions are in the form of small group teaching, generally with no more than one machine and instructor for a maximum of five students. The models/patients include normal models and patients with demonstrable pathology (e.g. peritoneal dialysis patients, patients with known abdominal aortic aneurysm).

A course manual is provided to help guide the student before the actual course. The course content generally covers the following topics:

- US physics
- instrumentation and image acquisition
- artefacts
- focused abdominal sonography in trauma (FAST): overview, anatomy, pathological findings
- abdominal aortic aneurysm (AAA): anatomy, pathology, measurement
- procedural US (such as central venous access, localization of a foreign body (FB)).

Many courses offer a pre- and post-course test (e.g. multiple choice questions) to confirm acquisition of core knowledge. Upon successful completion of the course, candidates usually receive a certificate of attendance.

Attendance at an introductory course is not a licence to practise US independently. Such courses are designed to introduce practitioners to the concepts and skills necessary for limited US.

 Attendance at an introductory course does not confer the experience and training required to practise US independently.

Advanced emergency US course

There is a wide range of available courses, from short university courses to masters level degrees. Courses differ in duration and content. The content may be similar to an introductory course but is of much greater depth and studied over a greater duration. Topics include those noted above and may include additional areas such as:

- deep vein thrombosis (DVT)
- emergency obstetric US, for example, ectopic pregnancy
- emergency echocardiography
- renal, for example, hydronephrosis
- musculoskeletal US
- testicular US.

Many courses consist of a lecture programme, directly supervised practice, indirectly supervised practice, course work and a final assessment of core knowledge and skills. The final assessment is more rigorous than that for introductory courses and may include US examinations carried out under real-time supervision and a written examination.

Unlike introductory courses, advanced courses *are* designed specifically to allow independent practice by successful candidates.

Credentialing

This is the process of acquiring the skill of reproducibly performing emergency US examinations to a predefined level. The routine use of US by non-radiologists such as cardiologists and obstetricians is not new. Emergency US has steadily grown in popularity and acceptance internationally and there is broad agreement that it should be part of normal daily practice.

It is the individual's responsibility to ensure his or her training is adequate. Until that individual has reached minimum credentialing standards a suitably trained supervisor must review all US scans before they can be used to affect clinical decisions. Hence, minimum standards of training and practice are essential.

Broadly speaking, to be credentialed the emergency US practitioner should have:

- attended a formal course
- performed and recorded a requisite number of 'proctored' US scans, under the direct supervision of an individual suitably qualified to provide such supervision
- passed an exit assessment which demonstrates the candidate's competency at performing emergency ultrasound.

Some issues remain unresolved, or have a range of proposed solutions. Particular questions include:

- Which specialty should perform US for certain indications?
- How many scans are required for credentialing?
- How should 'directly supervised scans' be defined: real-time supervision or later review by the supervisor?
- Should images be stored digitally, as single-frame hard-copy or video?
- When is a non-radiologist (such as an emergency physician) credentialed to train others in limited US?
- Whose responsibility is training of non-radiologists in emergency US?

Many of these issues have faced other non-radiologist specialties which perform US, such as obstetricians and cardiologists. In emergency US, the response to these issues differs in different jurisdictions and is still evolving. Appendix 2 lists useful organizations in Australasia, the USA and the UK which have responsibility for credentialing in emergency US.

Skills maintenance

Continuous professional development (CPD) and maintenance of practical skills are essential for the emergency US practitioner. This should include:

- regular scans
- ongoing training
- regular audit.

As for initial credentialing, minimum standards vary between international bodies. For example, The Australasian College for Emergency Medicine (ACEM) recommends 3 hours of US training, 25 FAST scans and 15 aorta scans annually with bi-monthly audit.

The Royal College of Radiologists (UK) have updated their 1997 guidelines for ultrasound scanning by non radiologists. The new guidelines reflect a more competency-based curriculum.

Log books

As diagnosis and treatment will be based on their result, all emergency US examinations must be documented, ideally in a personal logbook as well as in the formal patient record. The minimum entry details should include:

- patient and sonographer details
- date and type of US examination performed
- scan findings and the sonographer's interpretation of those findings
- a clear action plan based on the result (Appendix 1, Useful paperwork).

From an educational, audit and best practice viewpoint the findings and interpretation should be compared to other clinical data (e.g. CT, operative note, formal radiologist US) and comment made as to whether the emergency scan findings were accurate.

Summary

→ National standards vary.
→ Needs vary among individual practitioners.
→ Courses vary in content and duration.
→ Credentialing and skills maintenance are dynamic not static processes.

 There is no learning without feedback and audit.

 Static islands of training such as 1-day courses are insufficient unless part of a tailored ongoing skills development plan.

Chapter 15

Setting up an emergency ultrasound service

Sean McGovern, Peter Thompson

Introduction

Ultrasound (US) is becoming more available as technology develops. Emergency medicine clinicians have developed US scanning for both diagnostic and interventional purposes. This takes the form of focused US, which clearly differs from the often complex diagnostic scanning performed by radiologists.

Steps in establishing an emergency diagnostic US programme

This chapter will advise on the following steps but, as always, take advice from relevant local/national/international clinicians at the time to help make your plan succeed. *Consult broadly* as these steps usually occur contemporaneously and so need careful consideration from the outset.

- Select lead individual(s).
- Determine the scope and context of emergency US practice.
- Obtain radiology agreement/understanding.

- Develop a plan for implementation including:
  - acquisition of machine
  - training and credentialing the lead person(s) and the group, and continual professional development (see Ch. 14: *Getting trained and staying trained*).

Select lead individual(s)

This should be the person with the strongest interest or the most experience, who should also be effective as a negotiator. It is the most crucial decision of all, because if this individual has the right ideas but the wrong approach s/he will fail and the opportunity will be missed. Much depends on timing and the lead individual's ability to take advantage of opportunities as they arise.

Essential qualities include:

- respected and regarded clinician
- effective communicator and listener
- good negotiator: the ability to obtain consensus among clinical and management colleagues is vital

- understanding of how US can assist obtaining departmental goals
- clear plan for US training and future practice developments.

S/he should be a full-time staff member so not affected by separate time pressures or training needs. If not a consultant, s/he will need close consultant supervision and support.

This individual needs to:

- be focused on quality assurance and patient-centred practice
- develop links with the Radiology Department
- develop links with other clinical groups (obstetrics, cardiology, gastroenterology, renal/urology, intensive care) who use US in their practice
- be comfortable with the use of US: be fully trained or at least have attended an introductory course and several sessions in radiology to understand the limitations of US.

The scope and context of emergency ultrasound practice in your department

First, understand the limited scope that you wish to introduce. Go for the 'low-hanging' fruit: widely accepted applications of focused US such as abdominal aortic aneurysm (AAA) and focused assessment with sonography in trauma (FAST). Leave the more complex applications for later when the practice is established within the department. Understand the following:

- US is a rapid and safe way of diagnosing emergency conditions and should be part of the initial assessment of the seriously injured patient.
- Emergency diagnostic US should initially be seen as a binary 'rule in not rule out' tool, particularly in the training phase when false-negative scans are more likely.
- The business case needs to incorporate:
  - clinical indications, risk and clinical governance issues
  - machine capital and revenue costs
  - training costs and impact on clinical service
  - impact on other clinical services/colleagues.
- Focused emergency US has clear 'added value' for the assessment of:
  - torso trauma with FAST
  - abdominal aorta in symptomatic patients
  - vascular access.

Gaining and maintaining radiology department support

It is essential to consult broadly and get radiologists to understand your perspective, the limited nature of the scan and the importance of focused US for improved patient care and quality of service provision. Radiology support will ensure that the introduction of focused US is safe and successful. For example, a gold standard (e.g. CT or formal US in the Radiology Department) will be required for comparison with focused US, particularly in the training period.

Radiology support can be helped with data. The business case development that looks at patient numbers, outcomes and cost plus impact analysis will demonstrate to your radiology colleagues that you have considered the options and that you are committed to an effective, quality-driven service that will not have any negative implications for their practice.

Identify a lead radiologist, ideally with US as a subspecialty interest and with similar characteristics to those outlined above. It is important to find common ground – neither you nor the radiologists want poor practice within the ED. It is essential for all to understand that quality underpins the service provision. Remember that the Radiology Department remains a powerful resource with regard to advice on machine purchase and training of ED sonographers and their support will make the process much easier.

Recognize the growing radiologist workload and that they are indeed victims of their success. Also ensure that they understand that you and your department will take responsibility for training of your doctors but that you'd like advice/support/guidance. Radiologists are already swamped with their clinical practice as well as training their own juniors so they are appropriately concerned about adopting more trainees.

Once you do start using focused US, share your experiences (good and bad) with your clinical and radiological colleagues. Develop either clinical or US meetings that allow for appropriate sharing of information as well as helping to support the education and training of staff.

Plan for acquisition of the ultrasound machine

First, confirm that the machine is needed:

- audit activity for trauma/abdominal pain/central lines
- document difficulties with current practice: for example, the 'dangerous dash' for CT scans in trauma/the complications with central lines/the missed abdominal aortic aneurysms
- provide a simple cost analysis of scans performed for patients
- provide a suggested 'impact analysis' on the use of US: for example, reduce confusion with radiology/reduce need for out-of-hours CT/increase clinician confidence in clinical assessment.

Now that you've confirmed that focused US would help: *what type of machine?*

- portable yet sturdy and resilient for the ED and multiple practitioner use
- trolley/cart-based or hand-held (Figs 15.1 and 15.2)? Both have their advantages. The authors prefer trolley-based machines for their security and greater space for transducers and image storage
- suitable transducers for trauma and vascular access
- reasonable cost: midrange system with good image quality
- adequate after-sales training/maintenance support
- trial the machines (based upon these criteria) from a range of companies.

143

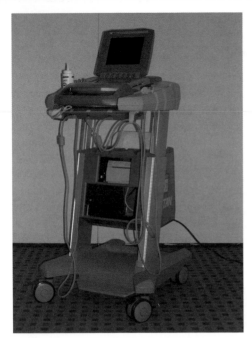

Fig. 15.1 Cart-based machine.

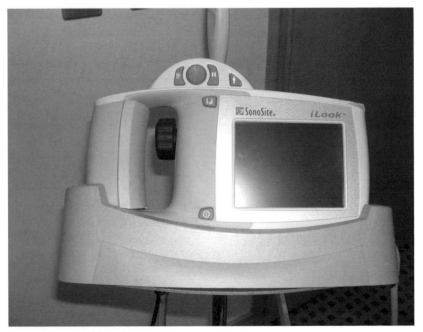

Fig. 15.2 Hand-held machine.

A machine business case requires early senior management support and understanding. Make the case in terms of activity and clinical governance and incorporate all obvious and hidden costs.

Summary

ED ultrasound is not new. It must be viewed in the context of a clinical adjunct aimed at improving the process for patients. A business case should be developed with a case mix of patients, capital cost of machine and ongoing revenue costs in mind. The ultrasound machine must be fit for the purpose: portable, lightweight, robust and with a facility to print or store images. Successful introduction requires ED ultrasound to complement rather than compete with radiologist-led scanning. A solid relationship should be maintained with a lead radiologist to facilitate the initial credentialing process. A lead ED physician should take forward matters relating to ED ultrasound and there should be regular teaching, audit and updates with respect to the same. Enthusiasm for use of ED-directed ultrasound must be tempered with knowledge of its limitations.

Chapter 16

Conclusion

Russell McLaughlin, Justin Bowra

The authors hope that you have found this book enjoyable and instructional. It cannot be stressed enough that:

- This book does not represent an exhaustive text of US. However, the reader should bear in mind that the clinician-US user does not require an exhaustive knowledge of all aspects of ultrasound.
- While this book represents one approach to the role of emergency US, this may not be the only valid approach.

The Emergency Sonographer simply requires the knowledge and skills required to answer the binary questions relating to a number of clinical questions. The aim of this chapter is to summarize the main areas which should be addressed when considering emergency point of care US on an individual and departmental basis.

Clinical

Based upon this book and the recommended training, these are the following questions the user should be asking:

Is there an abdominal aortic aneurysm?
Is there pleural fluid?
Is there pericardial fluid?

Is there free abdominal fluid?
Is there an above-knee deep vein thrombosis?
Is there a hip effusion?
Is the cannula in the correct vessel/fluid collection?
Is there a soft-tissue foreign body?
Is there evidence of cholelithiasis?
Is there hydronephrosis?
Is there an intrauterine pregnancy?

These questions should be answered only by yes/no/don't know. Straying beyond this or into other clinical questions without training represents dabbling, which is always dangerous. If you don't know or you need to answer a different question you need a radiologist.

Audit/quality control/training

The authors recommend that the practice of point-of-care emergency US is learned and practiced in a formal and structured manner including:

Audit and quality control

All US images should be reviewed for diagnostic quality and correct patient disposal on a regular basis. Ideally, this should occur as a joint exercise between the lead clinician in the ED and a radiology colleague.

Training

All clinicians engaged in training should be enrolled in a structured programme including supervised US practice, lectures and ideally an exit examination. This process is by no means standardized; however, it is the responsibility of the practitioner to agree on and achieve an acceptable standard of practice in keeping with local policy where national policy does not exist.

Managerial

It is the responsibility of the lead clinician/departmental manager to consider the broader issues relating to point-of-care ultrasound in the ED. These are as follows:

- Political. The most important issue here is the relationship with the Radiology Department. It is also vital that other stakeholders in the new service are aware of its limitations and benefits. It is vital that surgical colleagues are prepared to act on information given, e.g. AAA, abdominal fluid and hip effusion.
- Capital and revenue costs, including business case development for US machine.
- Audit/quality control/training. The department manager must ensure that all of these issues are addressed and that patient safety is paramount at all times.

Research and future directions

Like all areas of clinical practice it is important for clinicians to keep abreast of research and future developments in their own field and to implement evidence-based practice. Some clinicians may wish to engage in research and use point-of-care US as a useful tool.

Even though the technology is not new, the application of point-of-care US to certain emergency departments is very new. For example, evolving applications for ED US include testicular US and ocular US.

This concept of old technology–new application has driven many researchers to examine the use of US in the ED. Research projects involving bedside US can be used as a means of assessing the local applicability of a certain examination. For example, it may be possible to examine the impact of ED US on time to theatre in AAA patients who previously would have had Radiology Department examinations prior to theatre.

Research regarding ED US can be stratified into a number of levels:

- Technological/cutting edge, for example improved computer technology, US contrast, smaller US machines, 3-D US. It is likely that this research will come from the US manufacturers and research radiologists/scientists. There will probably be a significant lag phase of years before any useful ED application evolves.
- Clinical trials, for example FAST, AAA. There is good research from a number of centres worldwide on the benefits of these applications in the ED. However, users must first critically appraise the evidence in terms of their own local setting.
- Local validation studies, for example introducing a new application such as first-trimester scanning, biliary scanning. There is a role for introducing new applications based on evidence from other centres.

Summary

In summary, all of the above issues must be considered before embarking on ED US practice. The practitioner must be aware of the clinical and political issues and place the clinical condition of the patient above all. ED US will never replace sound clinical judgement.

 A fool with a stethoscope will still be a fool with an ultrasound.

Useful paperwork: logbook sheet

Sample ED ultrasound log

Adapted with permission from Emergency Department, Royal North Shore Hospital, Sydney, Australia

---

ED Ultrasonographer (name & signature)..........
....

Date & time..

Indication: ☐ Trauma   ☐ DVT
               ☐ Suspected AAA ☐ Other
               ☐ Vascular access

Patient's details (or apply sticker)

Details:...

Views: (tick as appropriate)	yes	no	Poorly visualized
Free fluid in Morison's Pouch	☐	☐	☐
Free fluid in Lienorenal angle	☐	☐	☐
Free fluid on suprapubic view	☐	☐	☐
Pericardial fluid	☐	☐	☐
Right ventricle abnormal	☐	☐	☐
Lung bases-pleural fluid	☐	☐	☐
Abdominal aortic aneurysm	☐	☐	☐
Deep venous thrombosis **above knee**	☐	☐	☐
Hip effusion on left	☐	☐	☐
Hip effusion on right	☐	☐	☐
Other eg FB (details)......................	☐	☐	☐

Images saved? ☐ Yes ☐ No

Hard Copy? ☐ Yes ☐ No **(please staple to this sheet)**

Ultrasound Diagnosis & time made: ....

Final Clinical Diagnosis & time made: ....

Basis of Final Diagnosis (eg CT): ....

Radiologist Review: name .... date ....

Adequate Images? ☐ Yes ☐ No

If Yes, Correct Interpretation? ☐ Yes ☐ No

Other Diagnostic Procedures:

	Confirm diagnosis	Refute diagnosis	Comment
CT	☐	☐	
Operation	☐	☐	
Other (eg angiogram)	☐	☐	

Appendix 2
Useful organizations

Up-to-date credentialing and specialty-specific information and guidelines are available from the following organizations. This is by no means an exclusive or exhaustive list of contacts in emergency ultrasound.

United States of America
- American College of Emergency Physicians (ACEP)
  - www.acep.org
- American College of Radiology (ACR)
  - www.acr.org
- American Institute of Ultrasound in Medicine (AIUM)
  - www.aium.org

Australasia
- Australasian College for Emergency Medicine
  - www.acem.org.au
- Australasian Society for Ultrasound in Medicine (ASUM)
  - www.asum.com.au

United Kingdom
- British Association for Emergency Medicine
  - www.baem.org.uk
- British Medical Ultrasound Society
  - www.bmus.org
- Royal College of Radiologists
  - www.rcr.ac.uk

Further reading

Beebe HG, Kritpracha B 2003 Imaging of abdominal aortic aneurysm: current status. Annals of Vascular Surgery 17:111–118.

Brenchley J, Sloan JP, Thompson PK 2000 Echoes of things to come: ultrasound in UK Emergency Medical Practice. Journal of Accident and Emergency Medicine 17:170–175.

Broos PLO, Gutermann H 2002 Actual diagnostic strategies in blunt abdominal trauma. European Journal of Trauma 2: 64–74.

Burnett HC, Nicholson DA 1999 Current and future role of ultrasound in the Emergency Department. Journal of Accident and Emergency Medicine 16:250–254.

Dart RG, Kaplan B, Cox C 1997 Transvaginal ultrasound in patients with low beta-human chorionic gonadotrophin values: how often is the study diagnostic? Annals of Emergency Medicine 30(2):135–140.

Durston W, Carl ML, Guerra W 1999 Patient satisfaction and diagnostic accuracy with ultrasound by emergency physicians. American Journal of Emergency Medicine 17(7):642–646.

Feigenbaum Harvey 1994 Echocardiography, 5th edn. Lea & Febiger, Baltimore, ISBN 0 8121 1692 5.

Hagen-Ansert Sandra L 1989 Textbook of diagnostic ultrasonography, 3rd edn. Mosby. ISBN 0 8016 2446 0.

Heller M, Jehle D 1997 Ultrasound in emergency: out of the acoustic shadow. Annals of Emergency Medicine 29:380–382.

Holmes JF, Harris D, Baltiselle FD 2003 Performance of abdominal ultrasonography in blunt trauma patients with out of hospital or emergency department hypotension. Annals of Emergency Medicine 43(3):354–361.

Jolly BT, Massarin E, Pigman EC 1997 Colour Doppler ultrasonography by emergency physicians for the diagnosis of acute deep venous thrombosis. Academic Emergency Medicine 4:129–132.

Kaddoura Sam 2002 Echo made easy. Churchill Livingstone, Edinburgh, ISBN 0 443 06188 2.

Kuhn M, Bonnin RL, Davey MJ et al 2000 Emergency department ultrasound scanning for abdominal aortic aneurysm: accessible, accurate, and advantageous. Annals of Emergency Medicine 36(3):219–223.

Lanoix R, Baker WE, Mele JM, Dharmarajan L 1998 Evaluation of an instructional model for emergency ultrasonography. Academic Emergency Medicine 5(1):58–63.

Ma O John, Mateer James R 2003 Emergency ultrasound. McGraw-Hill, New York, ISBN 0 07 137417 5.

Ma OJ, Mateer JR, Ogata M et al 1995 Prospective analysis of a rapid trauma ultrasound examination performed by emergency physicians. Journal of Trauma 38(6):879–885.

Mandavia DP, Aragona J, Chan L 2000 Ultrasound training for emergency physicians – a prospective study. Academic Emergency Medicine 7(9):1008–1014.

Mateer J, Valley V, Aiman E et al 1996 Outcome analysis of a protocol including bedside endovaginal sonography in patients at risk for ectopic pregnancy. Annals of Emergency Medicine 27:283–289.

McMinn RMH 1994 Last's anatomy, 9th edn. Churchill Livingstone, Edinburgh. ISBN 0 443 04662X.

Nilsson A 2002 Knowledge of artifacts helps prevent errors. Diagnostic Imaging Europe December 25–29.

Royal College of Radiologists. Faculty of Clinical Radiologists. 2005 Ultrasound training recommendations for medical and surgical specialties. London.

Schlager D 1997 Ultrasound detection of foreign bodies and procedure guidance. Emergency Medicine Clinics of North America 15:895–912.

Shih CHY 1997 Effect of emergency physician-performed pelvic sonography on length of stay in the Emergency Department. Annals of Emergency Medicine 29:348–352.

Sirlin CB, Brown MA, Deutsch R et al 2003 Screening ultrasound for blunt abdominal trauma: objective predictor of false negative findings and missed injury. Radiology 229: 766–774.

Taylor Kenneth JW 1985 Atlas of obstetric, gynecologic and perinatal ultrasonography, 2nd edn. Churchill Livingstone, Edinburgh, ISBN 0 443 08443 2.

Index